W0414992

AWTANI

Savoring Middle Eastern Homelands

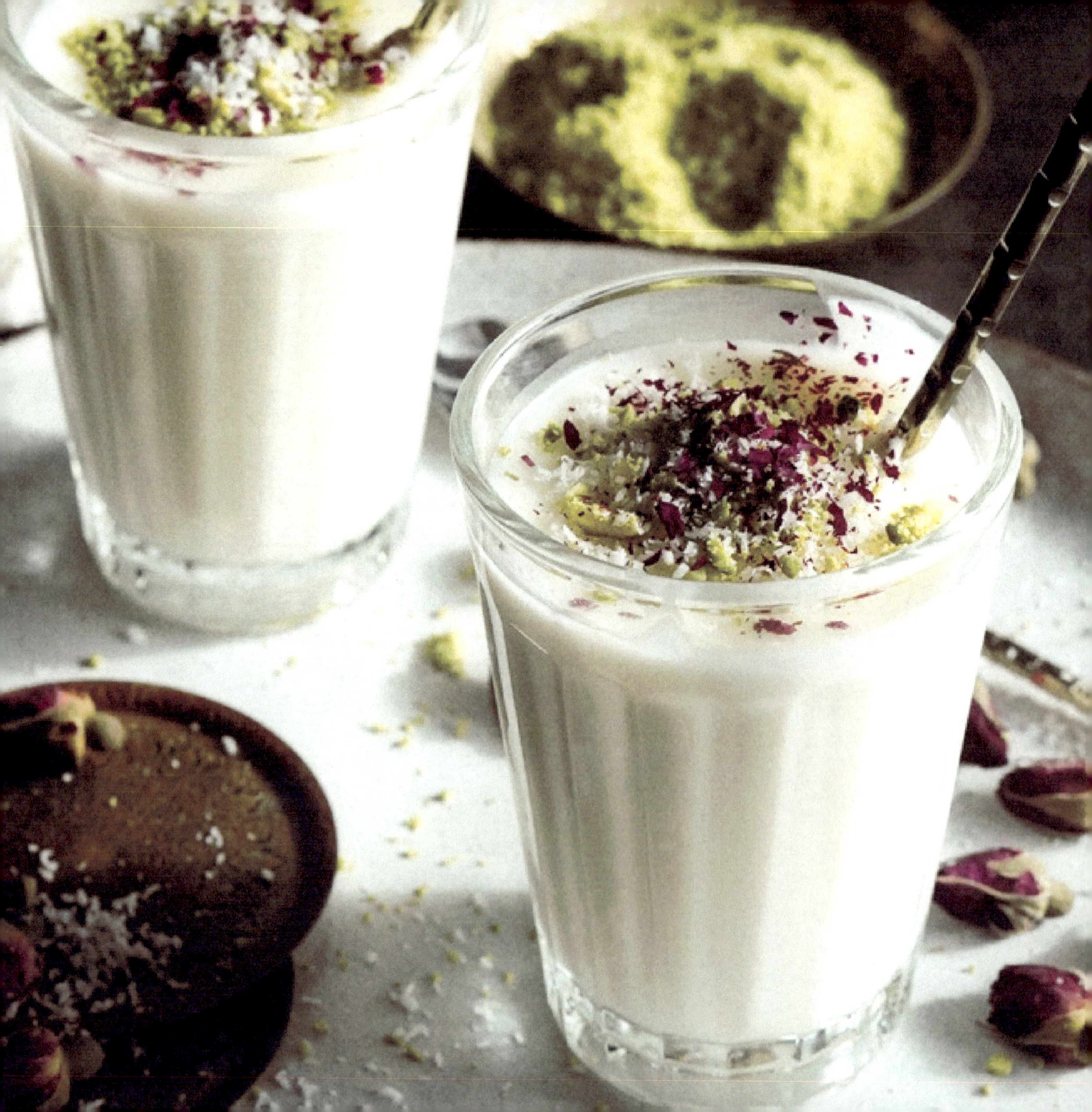

AWTANI

Savoring Middle Eastern Homelands

أوطاني

Fatimah M.A

Creator of Falasteenifoodie

Photography by Fatimah M.A

Copyright © 2024 Fatimah M.A

First published in 2024 by Fatimah M.A (Self-published)
www.Falasteenifoodie.com
Falasteenifoodie@gmail.com
Champaign, Illinois 61822

All rights reserved. No part of this book may be reproduced or used, in any form or by any means, electronic or mechanical, without prior permission in writing from Fatimah M.A.

ISBN: 979-8-218-36623-0

ISBN: 979-8-218-37043-5

Photography by Fatimah M.A

Edited by Rana Fakhereddin

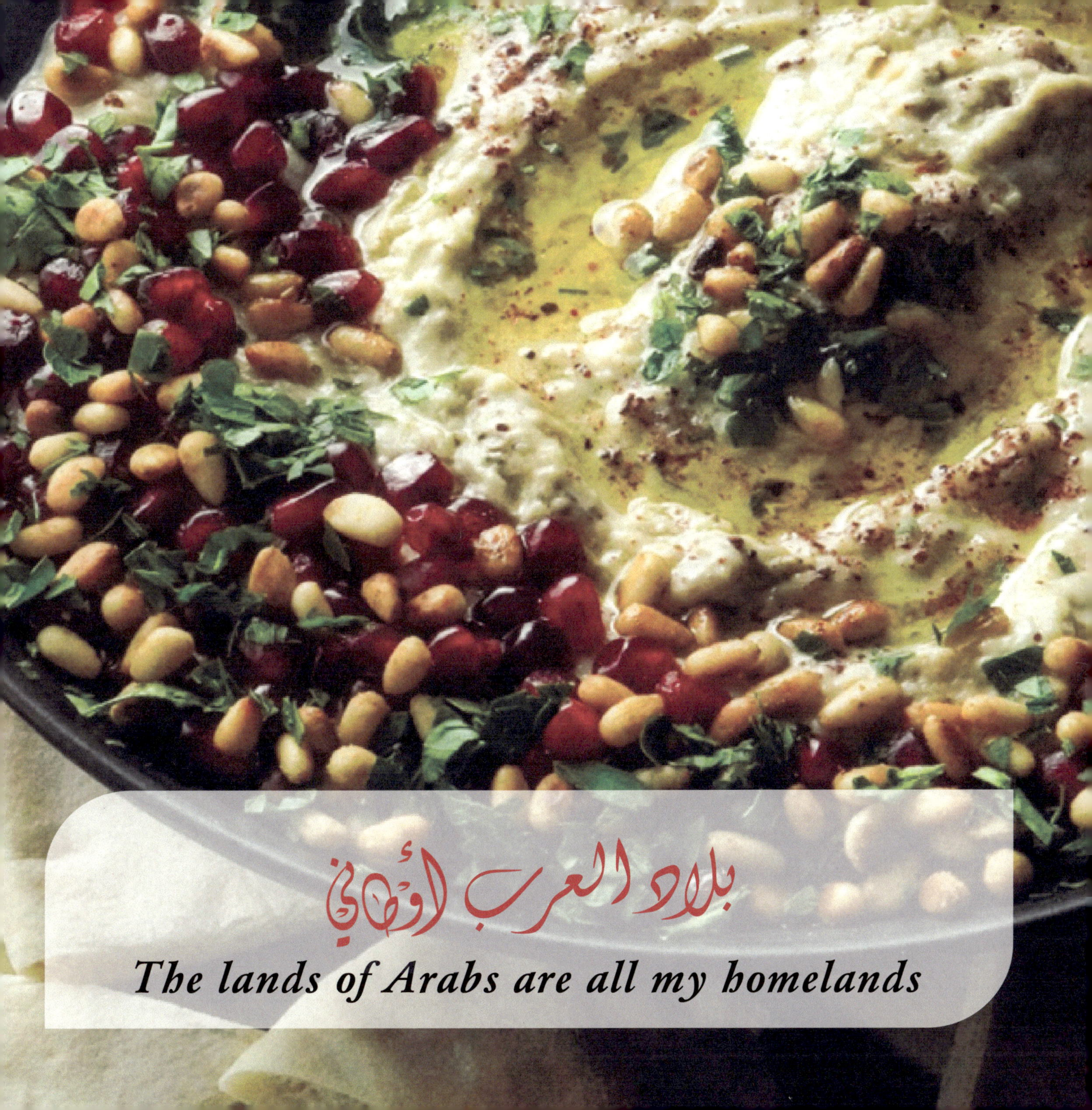
بلاد العرب أوطاني
The lands of Arabs are all my homelands

Table of contents

Introduction

Growing up in the heart of Amman during the early 2000s feels like flipping through a cherished photo album. Our little neighborhood was a colorful mosaic, mostly filled with Palestinians in the diaspora. Our humble abode may have been small, but it was bursting with life, a vibrant blend of Palestinian and various other cultures.

You see, we had this unique culinary fusion going on. Thanks to our earlier stint in the U.S., we were privy to a buffet of different dishes. So, imagine this: my mom's mini pizzas were like magnets, drawing my brothers' friends over. And there was a queue forming, not just for her tacos and meatloaf, but for a slice of our own little "international" cuisine party.

Picture me at the tender age of seven, a kitchen explorer whipping up concoctions that involved chocolate spread and tea biscuits, creating impromptu cookie sandwiches. I'd take za'atar manakeesh and marry them with labaneh in a baking experiment, aiming for the best of both worlds.

Now, let's talk about my mom, the unsung hero in our culinary escapades. Every Friday, like clockwork, she transformed our kitchen into a Maqlouba haven. But it wasn't just about Palestinian dishes. Nope, she dabbled in Kabsa and spiced up breakfast with Dibis and Tahina from the Arabian Gulf. A culinary world tour right at our dining table.

As I look back, I realize that despite our diverse dialects and varying traditions, Arabs from all corners share a profound love for cooking, hosting, and togetherness. We're united by our passion for good food and good company.

Yet, this unity comes with a bittersweet side. It means sharing not only joyous moments but also similar pains, bound by history and adversity. As a Palestinian, I intimately know the ache of having my culture, people, and land under occupation, feeling the theft of my people's identity. It's a collective suffering, unable to return to our homes and our land.

Enter Awtani, a tribute to us, to you. Beyond the shared pain lies a reminder of our commonalities. Our food, culture, and language are threads weaving our similarities into a beautiful tapestry. The dedication to preserving our heritage, seen in every recipe, is what allows me to savor these flavors.

So, to all of you who keep your culture alive, thank you. Awtani isn't just about recipes; it's about connection. Despite the barriers, we're all part of the same flesh and blood, sharing a profound connection through the richness of our shared experiences.

Here's to finding our homelands safe and sound, ready to be rebuilt with devotion and oneness. May Awtani be a vessel that brings us closer, one delicious dish at a time.

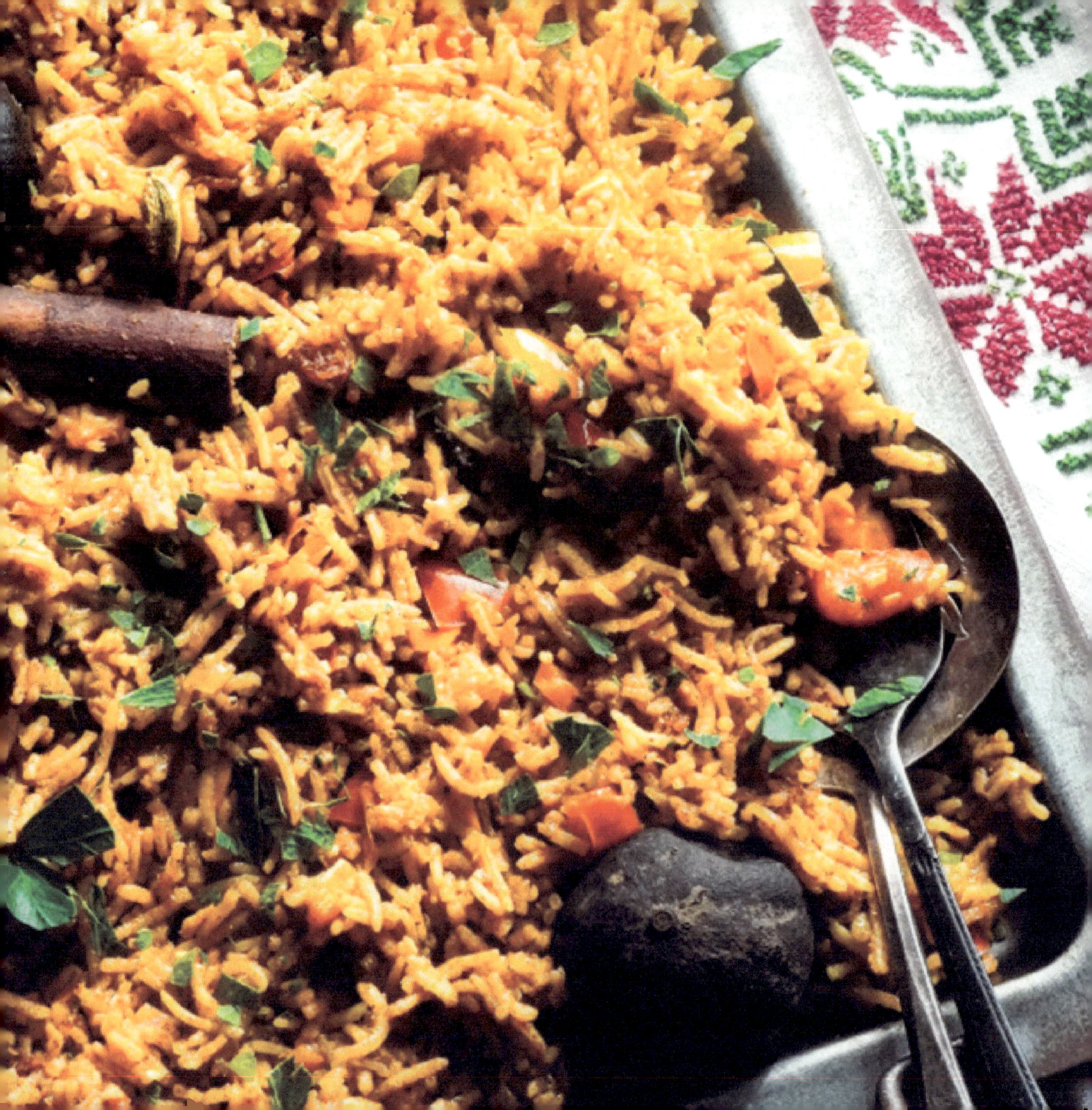

Ftour Arabi (Arab Breakfast)

فطور عربي

Arab breakfast, a delightful culinary journey that reflects the rich cultural tapestry of the Arab world, is a feast for the senses. Rooted in centuries-old traditions and influenced by diverse regional flavors, Arab breakfasts are a celebration of fresh ingredients, aromatic spices, and a warm sense of hospitality. From the indulgent pastries like Manakish to the sweet dibis and rashi, each morning meal tells a story of heritage and connection.

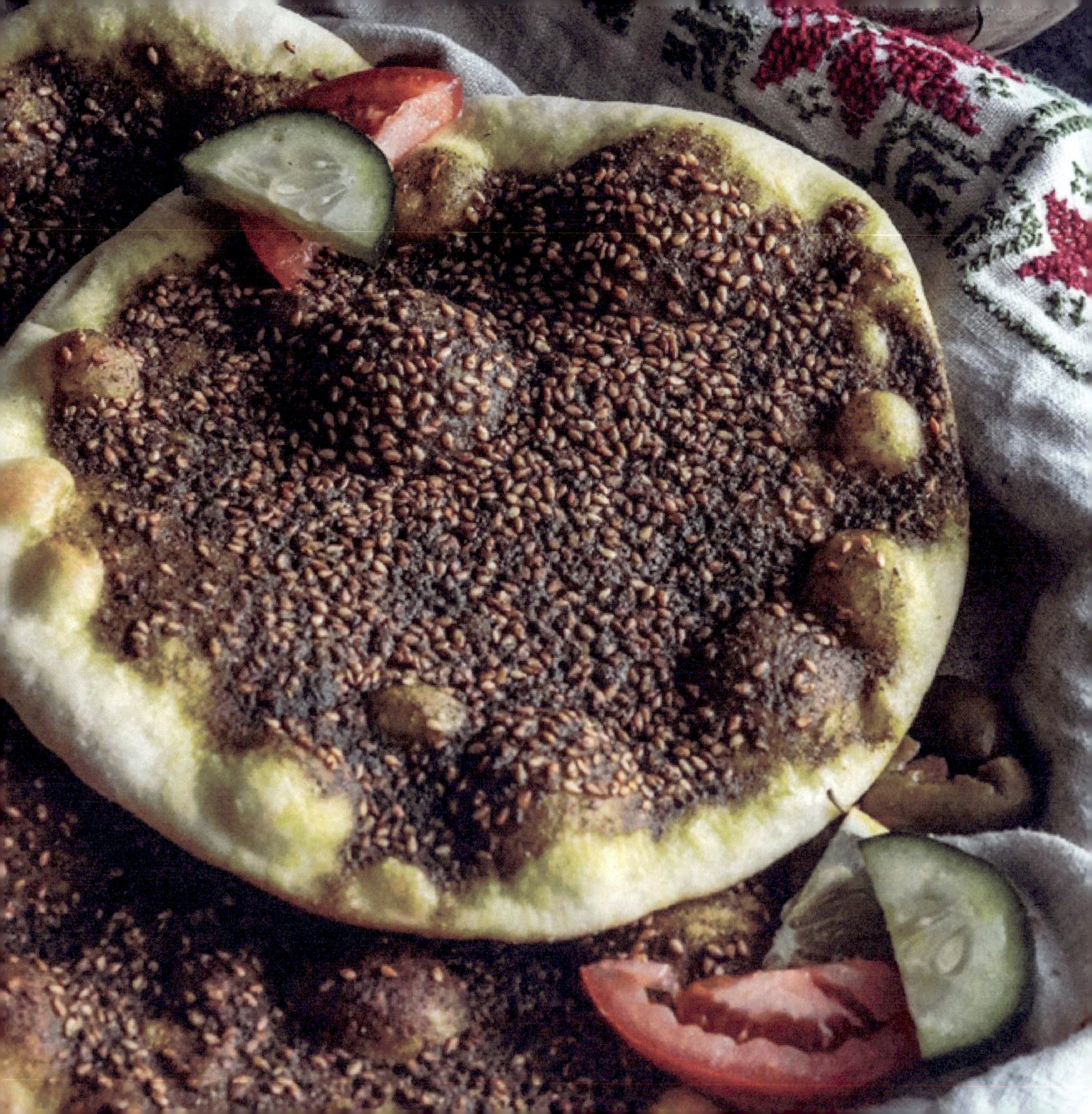

Batata Harra بطاطا حارة

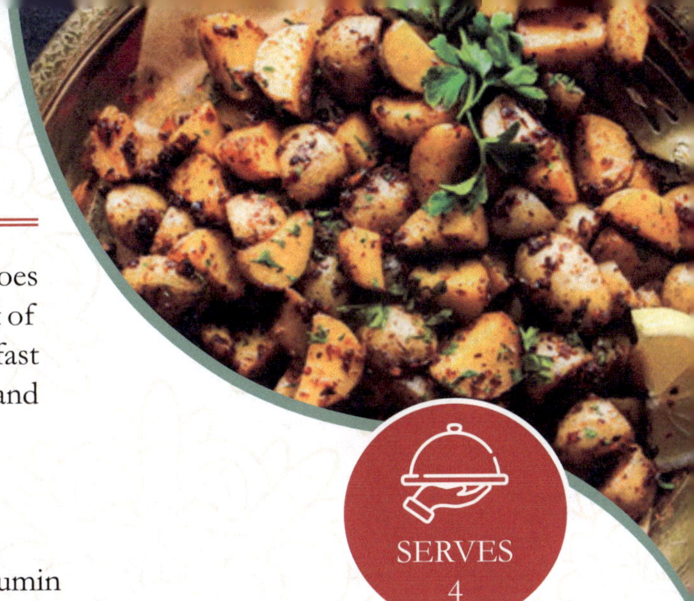

Batata Harra – a Middle Eastern dish that turns ordinary potatoes into a flavorful delight. This Middle Eastern classic brings a burst of spices to the humble potato. Whether you're after a tasty breakfast or a satisfying snack, these crispy spiced potatoes with garlic and chili are the way to go.

SERVES 4

INGREDIENTS:

- 1 lb baby potatoes, washed and quartered
- 3 tbsp extra virgin olive oil
- 5 garlic cloves, minced
- 1 tsp salt
- ¾ tsp 7 spices
- ½ tsp ground cumin
- 1 tsp Aleppo pepper, or to taste
- 1 ½ tbsp shatta (Middle Eastern Chili Paste)

DIRECTIONS:

1. Fill a large pot with water, and bring to a boil.
2. Wash the potatoes, and cut into quarters.
3. Add the potatoes to the pot of boiling water, and cook until fork tender. Drain and set aside.
4. In a separate skillet, heat up the olive oil on medium-high heat.
5. Add the minced garlic and saute until golden, about 3-5 minutes.
6. Add the boiled potatoes
7. Toss in the 7 spices, Aleppo pepper, shatta, cumin, and salt. Mix together well. Let it cook together for another minute or two and remove.
8. Serve with pita bread, as a breakfast side, or as a snack.

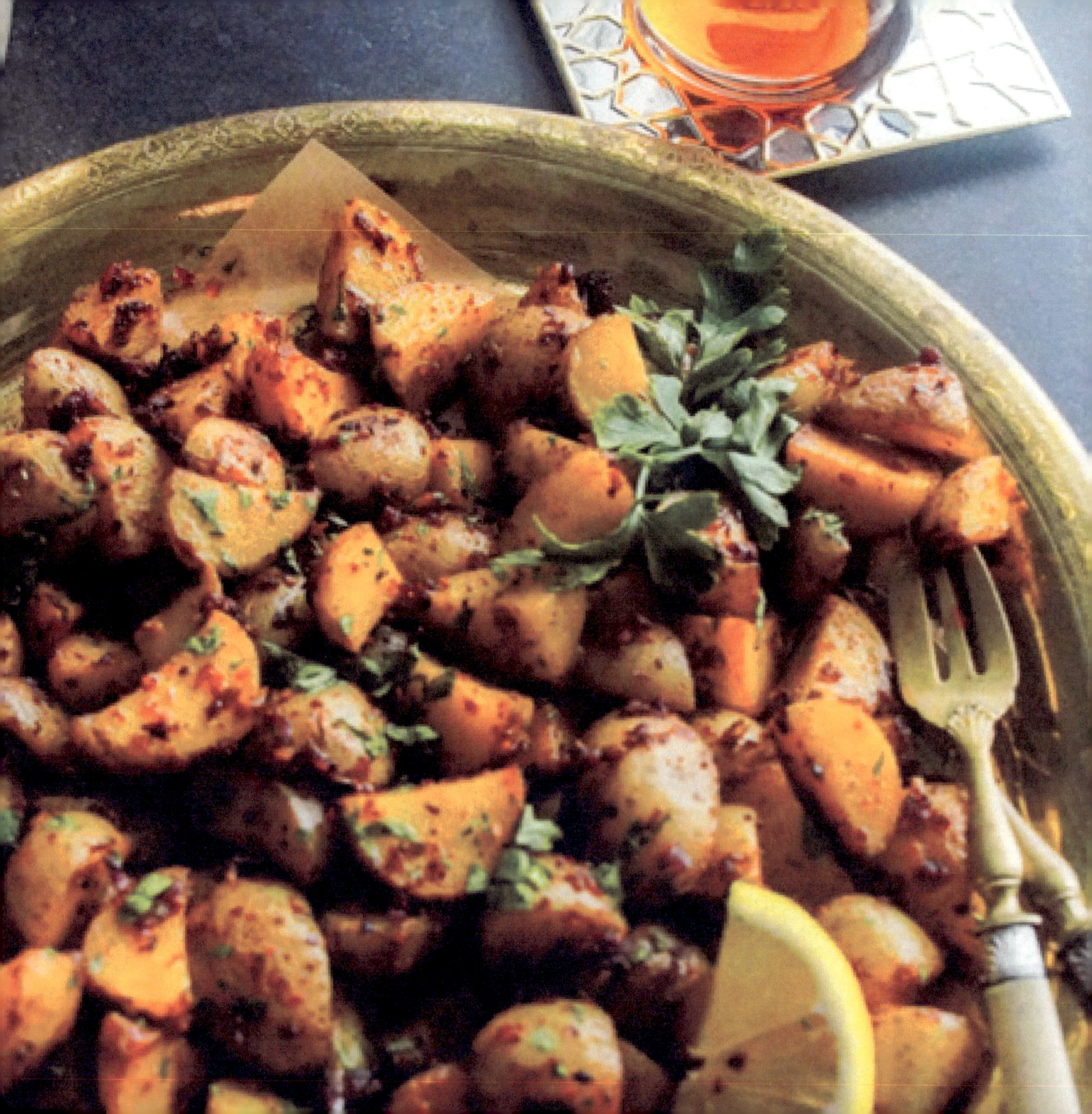

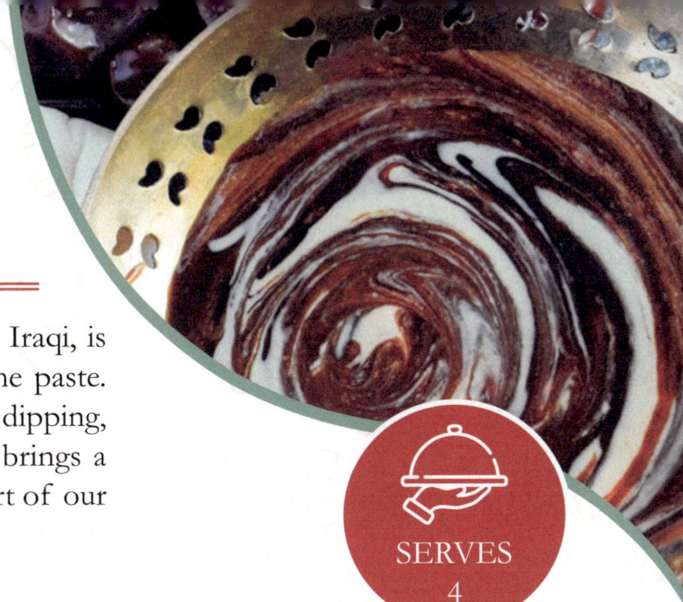

Dibis Ou Tahiniyeh

(Date Syrup and Tahini) دبس وطحينة

Dibis Ou Tahiniyeh, or Dibis and Rashi if you're Kuwaiti and Iraqi, is a Middle Eastern combo that's all about date syrup and sesame paste. This duo adds a unique flavor to your desserts, whether you're dipping, spreading, or drizzling. It's a simple and versatile combo that brings a taste of the Middle East to your table. We typically have it as part of our breakfast spread, or add it on top of cakes and desserts.

SERVES
4

INGREDIENTS:

- ½ cup date molasses
- ⅓ cup tahini
- Pinch of salt

DIRECTIONS:

1. Make sure to mix the tahini well so it isn't too oily.
2. Add the date syrup, tahini, and salt to a bowl. Mix together well with a whisk.
3. Enjoy with warm pita or use it to top cakes!

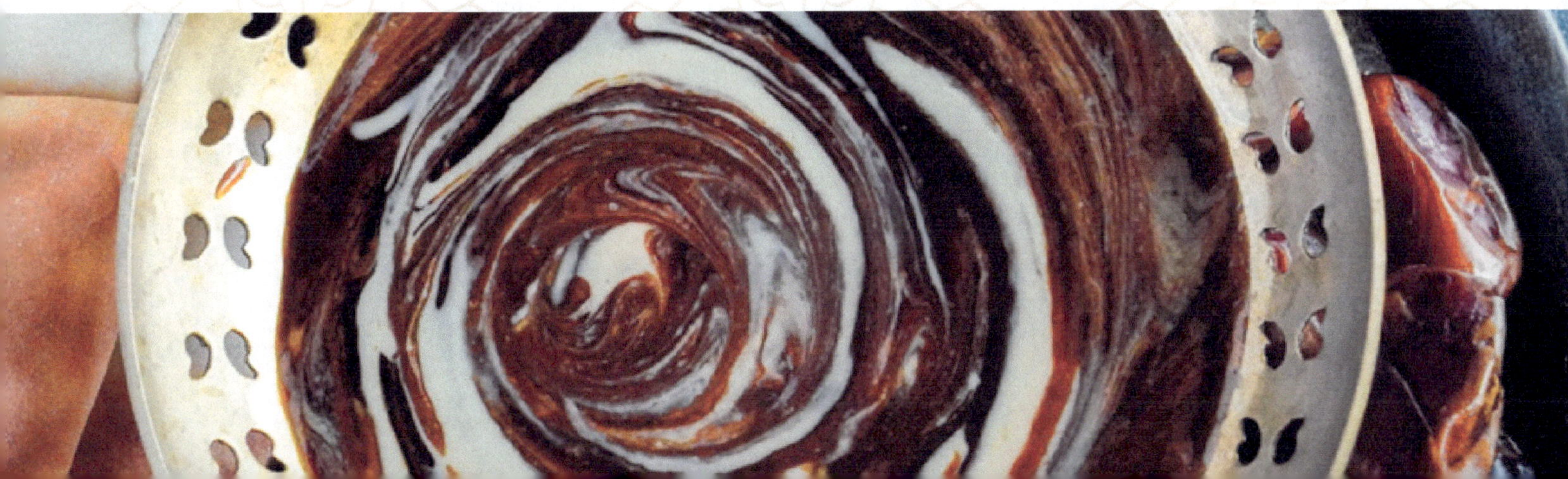

Qalayet Bandoora قلاية بندورة

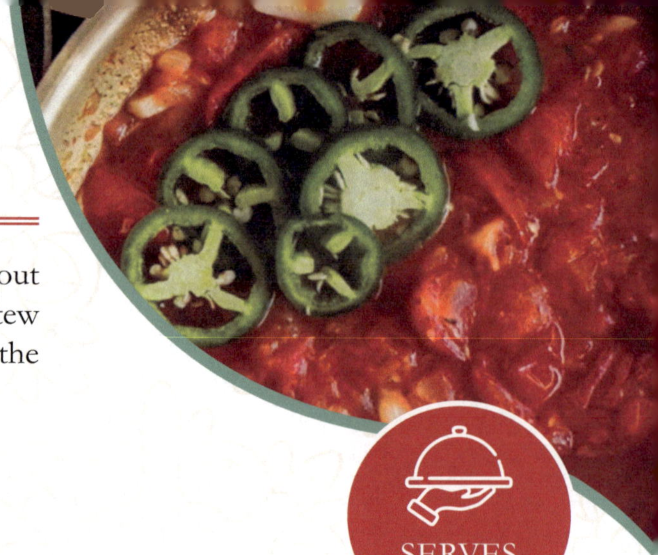

A Middle Eastern, more specifically Palestinian, dish that's all about tomatoes, garlic, and onions. This simple breakfast and brunch stew packs a punch of flavor with the goodness of ripe tomatoes, the savory kick of garlic, and the aromatic touch of onions.

SERVES 2-3

INGREDIENTS:

- 3 tbsp extra virgin olive oil
- 1 small yellow onion, finely chopped
- 5 garlic cloves, minced
- 4 large tomatoes, cut into medium sized cubes
- 1 tsp salt, or to taste
- ½ tsp black pepper
- Jalapenos, to taste

DIRECTIONS:

1. Heat a skillet on medium-high heat. Add in the olive oil and allow it to become hot.
2. Add in the finely chopped onions. If you're using jalapenos, add them here as well. Saute until the onions are a little fragrant, about 2-3 minutes.
3. Add the minced garlic and mix well. Let the aromatics saute for another 3-5 minutes until softened, and the garlic is golden.
4. Add in the chopped tomatoes.
5. Season with salt and pepper, and mix well.
6. Immediately lower the heat to medium-low, and cover the skillet.
7. Let this cook for 5-10 minutes, or until the tomatoes are completely jam-like and softened. Give everything one final stir and adjust the seasonings.
8. Serve with warm pita bread.

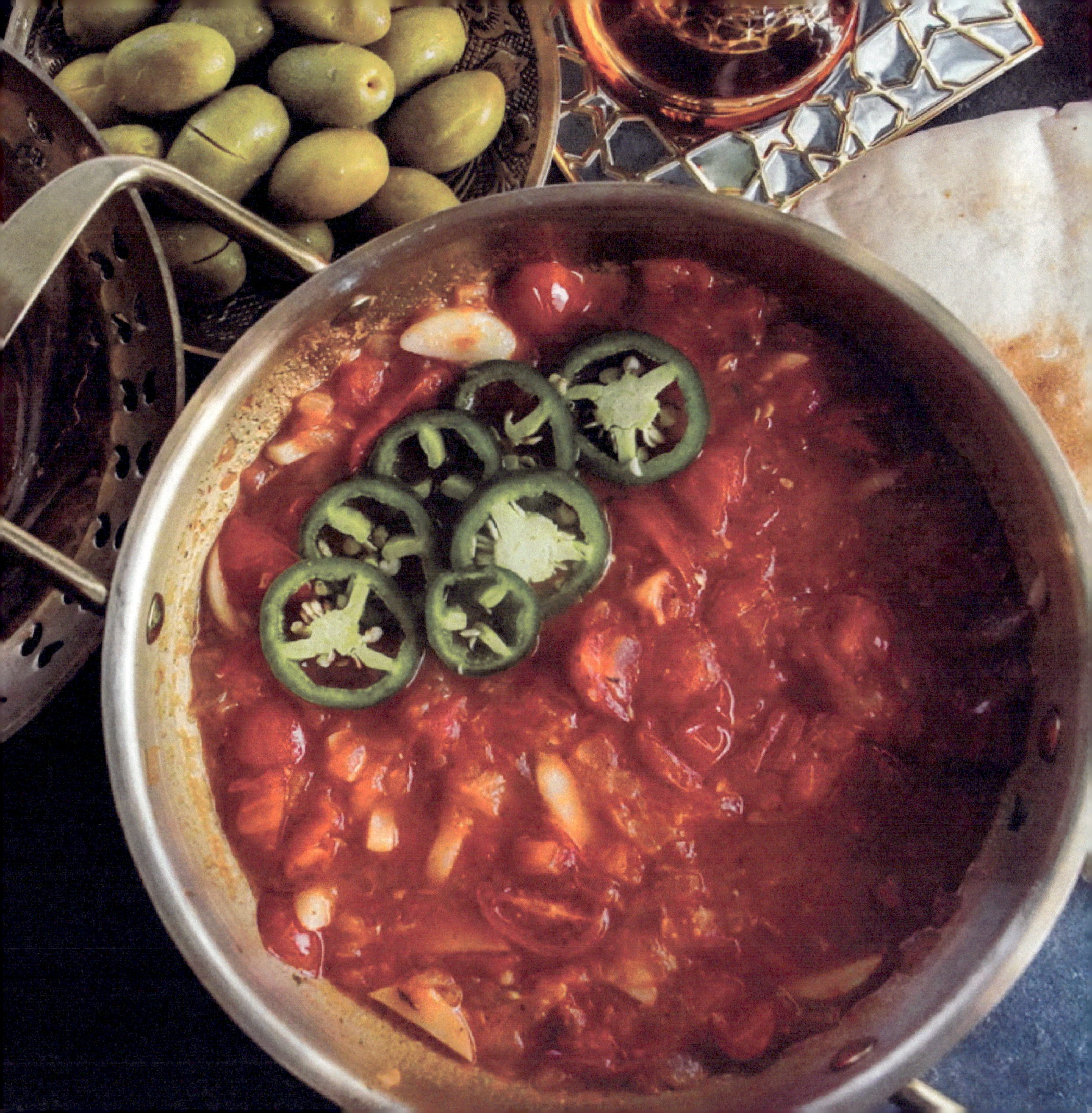

Mamounieh مامونية

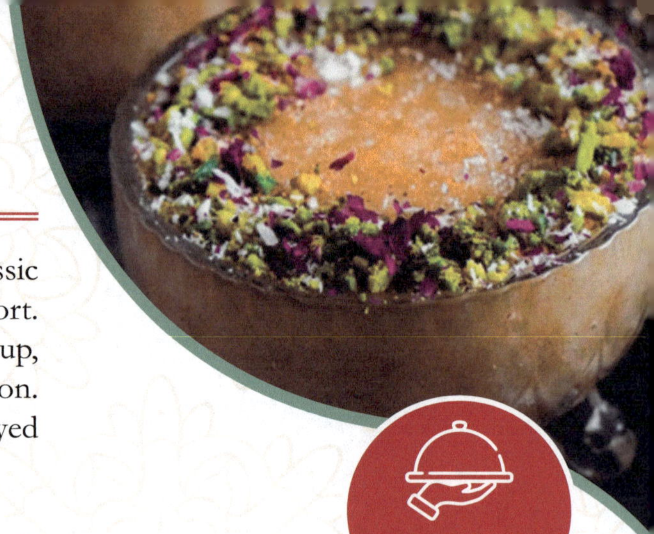

SERVES 4

Get ready for a taste of Syrian tradition with Mamounieh – a classic Middle Eastern dessert or breakfast that's all about simple comfort. This sweet treat, made with semolina and soaked in a sugary syrup, is topped off with a hearty sprinkle of pistachios and cinnamon. It's a straightforward and indulgent delight that has been enjoyed for ages.

INGREDIENTS:

- ⅓ cup granulated sugar
- 4 cups water
- 2 tbsp unsalted butter
- 2 tbsp ghee
- 1 cup coarse semolina
- ¾ tsp ground cinnamon
- 1 tsp rose water, optional

DIRECTIONS:

Prepare The Sugar Syrup:

1. In a saucepan, combine sugar and water.
2. Bring to a boil, stirring until the sugar dissolves.
3. Simmer for 5 minutes until it slightly thickens.
4. Stir in the rose water and set aside. Do not let the syrup completely cool down. Begin working on the semolina.

Toast Semolina:

1. In a separate pan, melt the butter and ghee over medium heat.
2. Add the semolina and stir continuously until it turns golden brown and gives off a nutty aroma. Be cautious not to burn it.
3. Gradually pour the sugar syrup into the toasted semolina, stirring constantly to avoid lumps.
4. Continue cooking over low heat until the mixture thickens.
5. Immediately transfer the Mamounieh mixture into 4 serving dishes, spreading it evenly.
6. Allow it to cool and set for a few minutes. It is best eaten warm.
7. Garnish with the remaining chopped nuts and a sprinkle of ground cinnamon if desired.

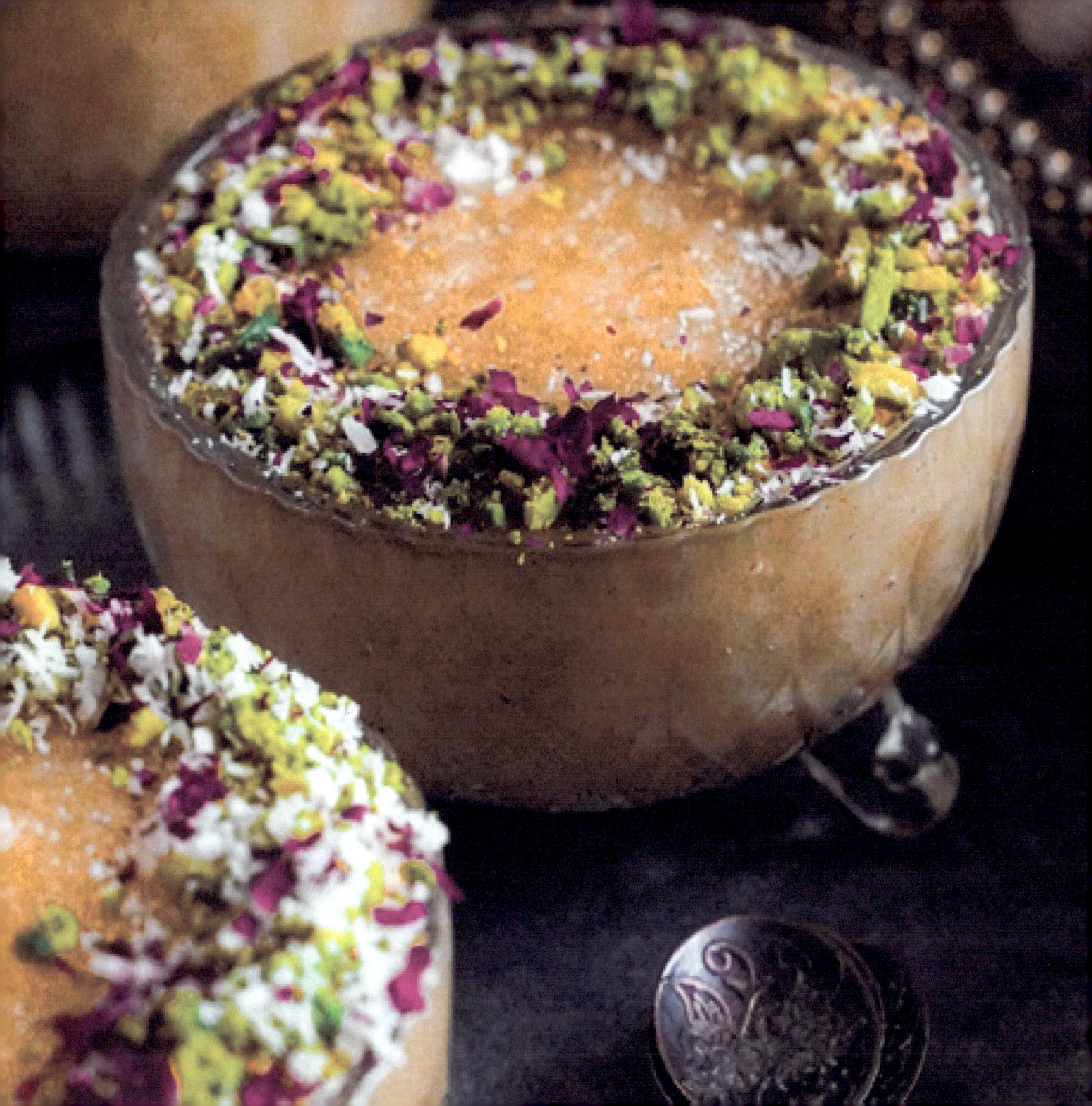

Za'atar Egg Salad سلطة بيض وزعتر

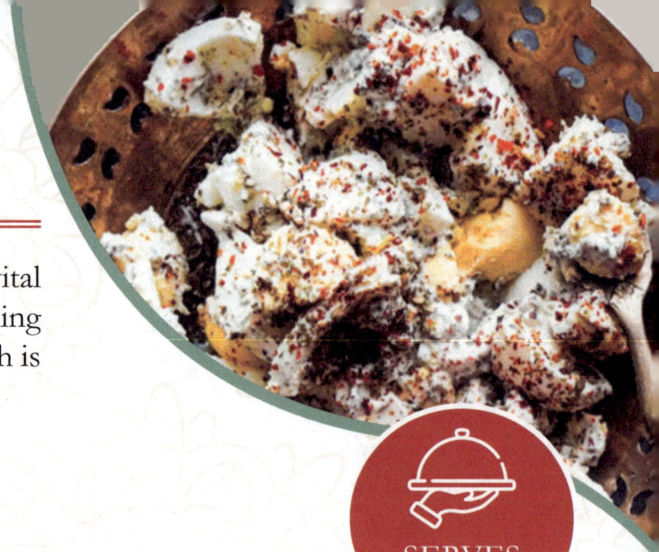

It is no surprise that both za'atar and eggs-both containing vital nutrients- are an essential part of an Arab breakfast, and combining them yields a tasty, delicious, and wholesome breakfast. This dish is comprised of a few different Arab breakfast staples.

SERVES 2-3

INGREDIENTS:

- 4 large eggs
- 2 tbsp labneh
- 1 tbsp extra virgin olive oil
- 1 tbsp za'atar
- ½ tsp Aleppo pepper
- ¼ tsp black pepper, or to taste
- ½ tsp salt or to taste

DIRECTIONS:

1. Begin by boiling the eggs. Place them into a large pot and ensure the water level is 2 inches above the eggs when covering them. Place them on high heat and let them boil for 11-12 minutes. You want these to be hard boiled. Once done, remove the eggs from the hot water and transfer them into cold water to allow for easy peeling.
2. Once the eggs are peeled, cut them into halves, then into quarters. Each egg should give about 8 pieces.
3. Add the cut up eggs into a bowl. Add the labneh, olive oil, and za'atar. Add the Aleppo pepper, salt, and black pepper and mix. You can mix in chopped tomatoes, Middle Eastern pickles, or olives if you'd like.

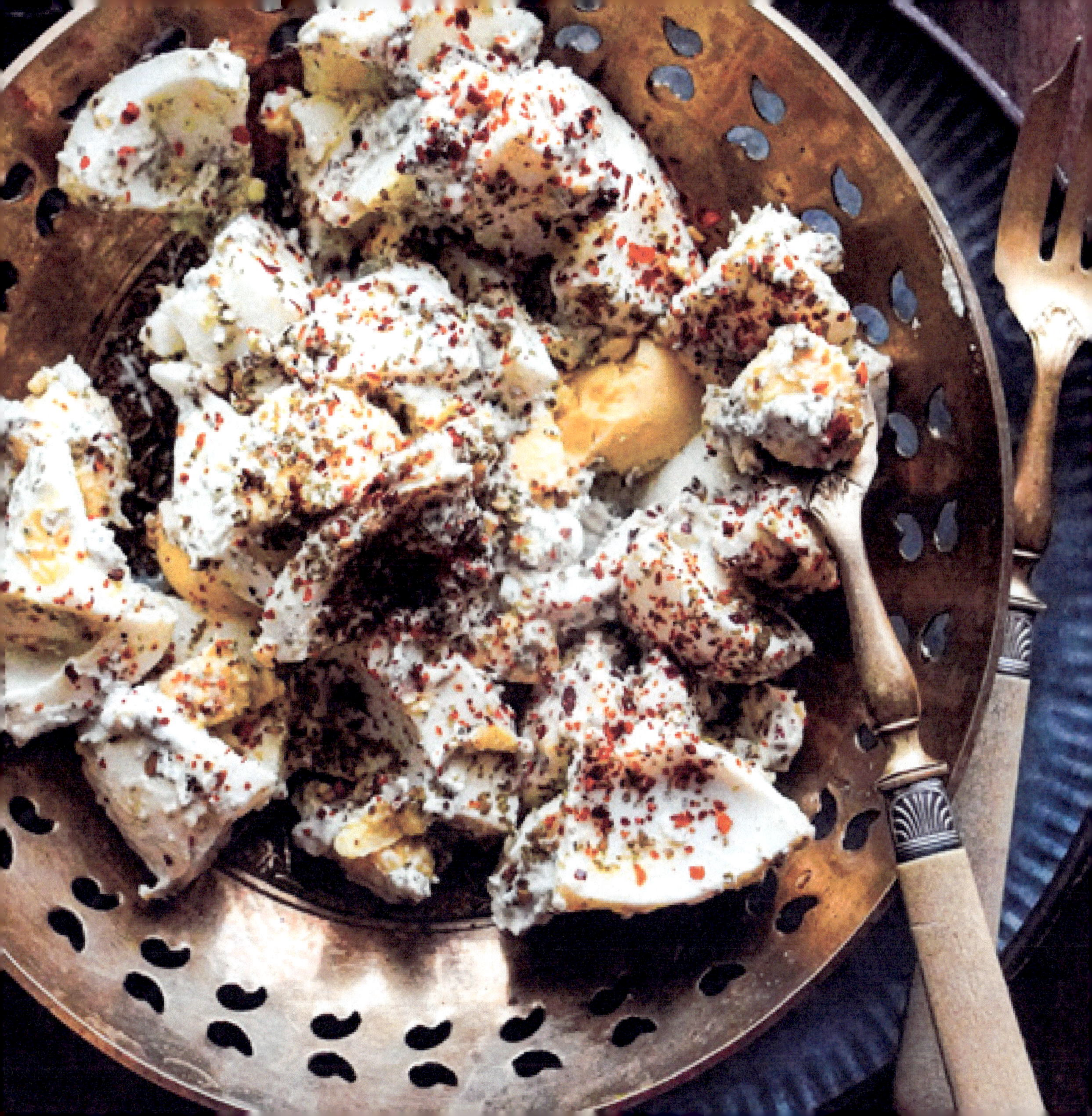

Za'atar Manakeesh مناقيش زعتر

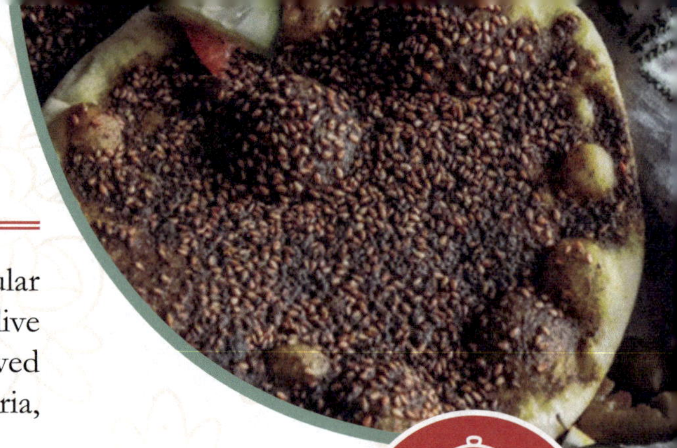

SERVES
8-12

Za'atar Manakeesh, also known simply as Manakeesh, is a popular Middle Eastern flatbread topped with a mixture of za'atar, olive oil, and sometimes other ingredients. It is a traditional and beloved dish in the Levant region, including countries like Lebanon, Syria, Jordan, and Palestine, which za'atar originated from.

INGREDIENTS:

Small Batch 10 Minute Dough:

- 2⅔ cups all purpose flour
- ¼ cup oil, extra virgin olive oil or any neutral oil
- ¾ tbsp active dry yeast
- 2 tsp granulated sugar
- ½ tsp salt
- ½ tsp baking powder
- 1 cup warm water or warm milk

Za'atar mix:

- 1 cup zaatar
- ¾ cup extra virgin olive oil

DIRECTIONS:

1. Preheat the oven to 450 F.
2. Mix 1 cup of flour with the yeast, sugar, salt, and baking powder.
3. Once mixed, add the warm water or warm milk, and whisk together well until no longer clumpy.
4. Cover and set aside in a warm place for 10 minutes. After 10 minutes, you should see the mixture look bubbly and frothy.
5. Now, add the remaining 1⅔ cup of flour and the oil.
6. Mix in your stand mixer, or by hand, until a smooth and soft dough forms, about 5-7 minutes.
7. Divide into 8 large pieces or 12 small ones, and let them rest for 2 minutes.
8. Line a baking sheet with parchment paper.
9. Roll each dough ball thinly.
10. Mix the zaatar and olive oil
11. Spread a generous amount onto each rolled out piece of dough, avoiding the edges.
12. Place onto the baking sheet and bake for 10-15 minutes, or until the dough puffs out slightly and has a golden color to it.

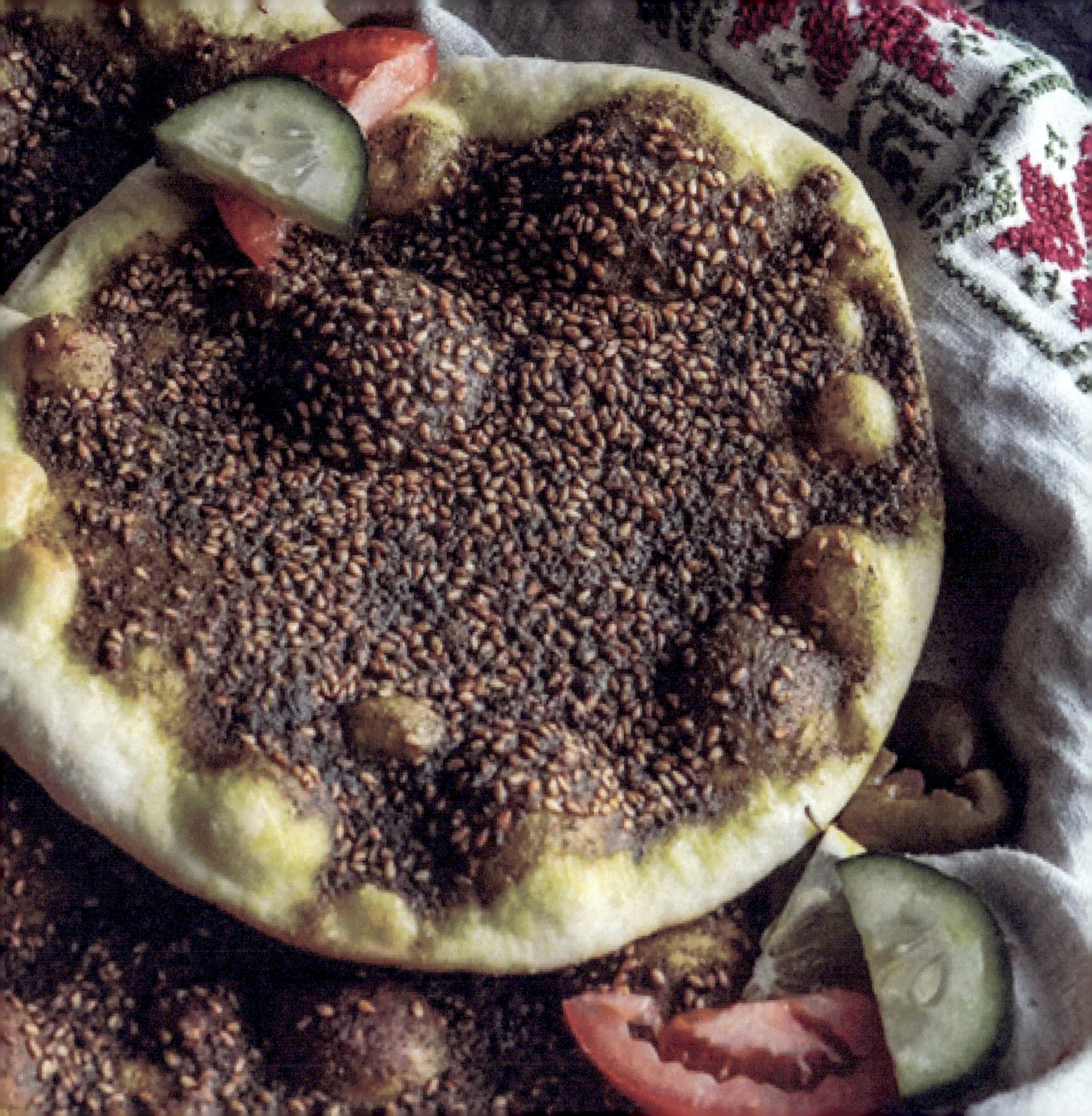

Muqabilat Arabiya (Arab Appetizers and Sides)

مقبلات عربية

Embark on a tantalizing journey through the world of Arab side dishes and appetizers, where every bite is a symphony of flavors that dance on your palate. Steeped in centuries of culinary history, Arab cuisine boasts an array of delectable starters and accompaniments that showcase the region's rich tapestry of tastes and aromas. From the savory delights of Mutabal to the crisp, golden perfection of Kubbeh, these dishes are a testament to the art of blending fresh, wholesome ingredients with a medley of aromatic spices. Whether enjoyed as a prelude to a main course or savored as a shared feast, Arab side dishes and appetizers promise an exquisite culinary experience that transcends borders and captivates the senses.

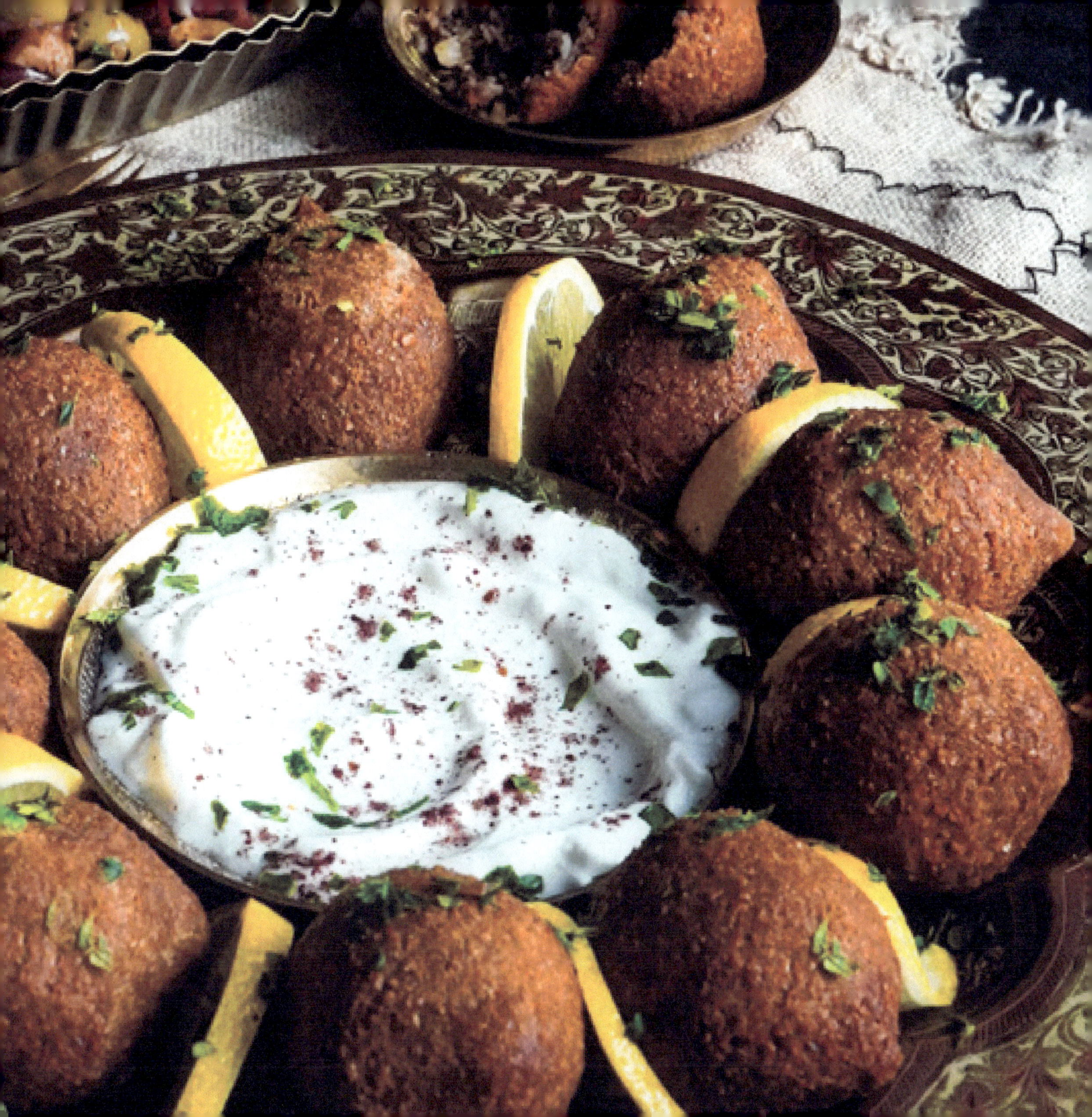

Fattet Arayes فتة عرايس

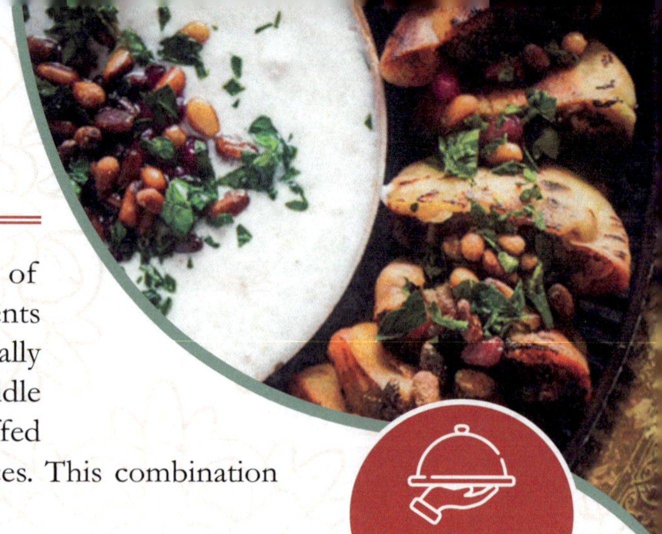

Fatteh is a traditional Middle Eastern dish that features layers of toasted or fried pieces of flatbread, topped with various ingredients that range from hummus, to eggplants and chicken, and is usually topped with a flavorful yogurt sauce. Arayes is a popular Middle Eastern Arab dish, and are essentially grilled or oven-baked stuffed pita sandwiches that combine ground meat with aromatic spices. This combination makes for a great appetizer or side dish at any dinner table.

SERVES 4

INGREDIENTS:

Arayes:

- ½ small yellow onion
- 1 roma tomato
- ¼ cup parsley leaves
- 4 garlic cloves
- ½ lb ground beef (best to use more lean beef, about 90%)
- 1 ½ tsp 7 spices
- ¼ tsp black pepper
- ¾ tsp salt, or to taste
- ¼ tsp Aleppo pepper
- 14 oz mini pita pockets (about 2 packages)
- 3 tbsp extra virgin olive oil

Garlic Yogurt:

- 5 garlic cloves
- 2 tbsp unsalted butter
- 1½ cups plain whole milk yogurt
- 1 tbsp lemon juice
- Salt, to taste
- ¼ tsp sumac
- 2 tbsp water

DIRECTIONS:

1. To prepare the arayes filling, begin by adding the onion, garlic, parsley and tomato to a food processor. Process until chunky, but not watery.
2. Add the ground beef to a bowl, and top with the vegetable mixture.
3. Add the 7 spices, black pepper, salt, and Aleppo pepper. Mix until well combined.
4. Take the mini pitas and cut them in half. Add a hefty amount of beef filling to each mini pita (about 1 ½ tbsp) and repeat until finished.
5. Heat up the olive oil on medium heat.

6. Add the mini pita halves meat side down, careful not to overcrowd the pan. Cook in batches if needed. Cook each one for 3-4 minutes, or until browned.
7. Flip the pitas around and brown on each side to ensure even cooking. You could also cover the pan to help steam them and ensure properly cooked beef.
8. To make the yogurt, start by melting the unsalted butter on high heat.
9. Add the minced garlic and saute until golden, about 2 minutes.
10. In a bowl, combine the fried garlic along with the butter in the pan and the yogurt.
11. Add the lemon juice, sumac, and salt to taste. Mix well.
12. Add the water to thin it out, and mix again.
13. To serve, add the yogurt dip to a bowl in the middle of a large platter.
14. Add the arayes halves all around the bowl to make a ring.

To serve, top the mini arayes with parsley, toasted pine nuts, and pomegranate seeds.

Pro Tip: I use the Joseph's Bakery mini pitas for ease, but you could use mini tortilla, or cut up a whole pita into small pieces.

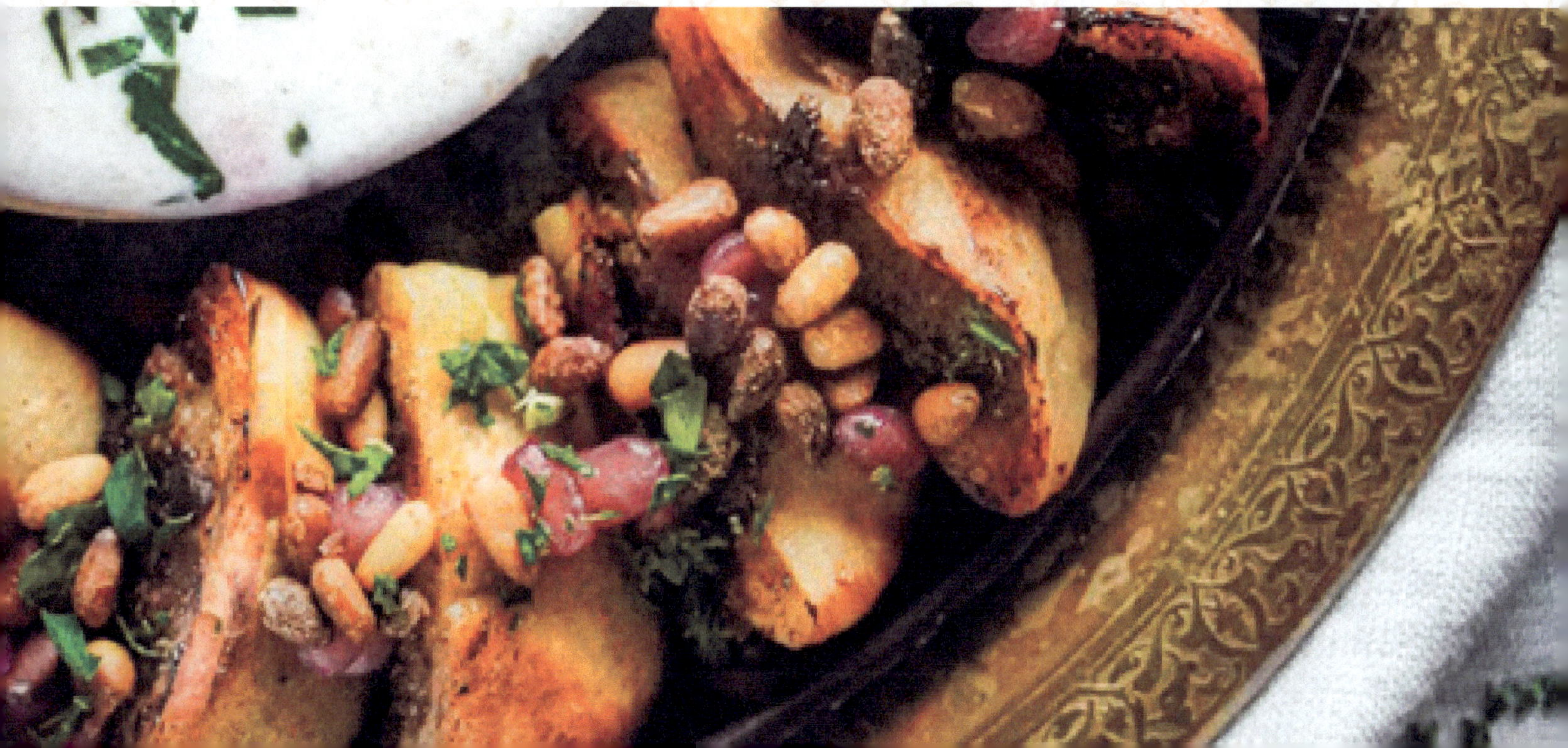

Mthawamet Batata مثومة بطاطا

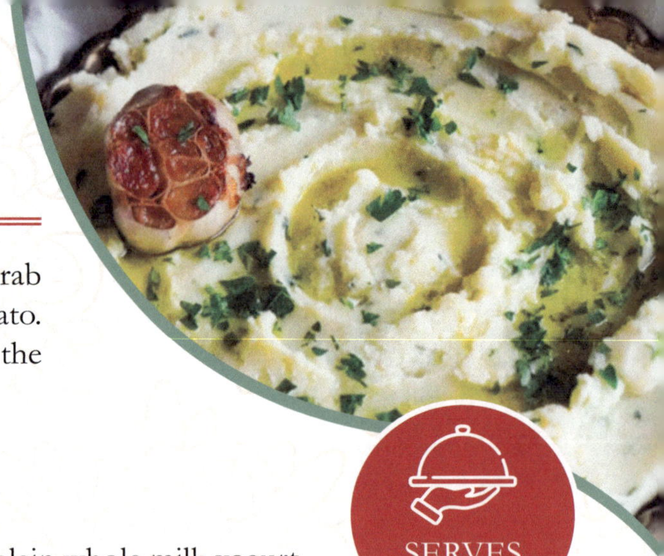

Mthawamet Batata is a mashed potato dish riddled with Arab flavors and twists. It slightly differs from the classic mashed potato. Its infused with extra virgin olive oil, yogurt, and parsley. This is the perfect side dish to accompany your Middle Eastern feasts.

SERVES
6-8

INGREDIENTS:

- 5 medium potatoes, peeled
- 10 garlic cloves
- 1/3 cup + 1 tbsp extra virgin olive oil ,divided
- 1/3 cup plain whole milk yogurt
- 1/3 cup chopped parsley
- 1 tbsp lemon juice
- Salt and pepper to taste

DIRECTIONS:

1. Preheat the oven to 400 degrees.
2. Peel and wash the potatoes. Enclose the potatoes in aluminum foil and seal them shut. Add to a baking sheet. Add the garlic cloves to a foil pocket and drizzle with 1 tsp olive oil. Then, seal shut and place on the baking sheet.
3. Bake for 30-40 minutes, or until the potatoes are fork tender and the garlic is gold and jam-like. Remove from the oven and let it cool.
4. Transfer the potatoes and garlic to a bowl and mash well. Add the olive oil and yogurt and mix together well. Add in the chopped parsley, lemon juice, and seasonings. Mix together well until everything is well incorporated.
5. Transfer to a serving dish and top with another drizzle of olive oil and some more chopped parsley.

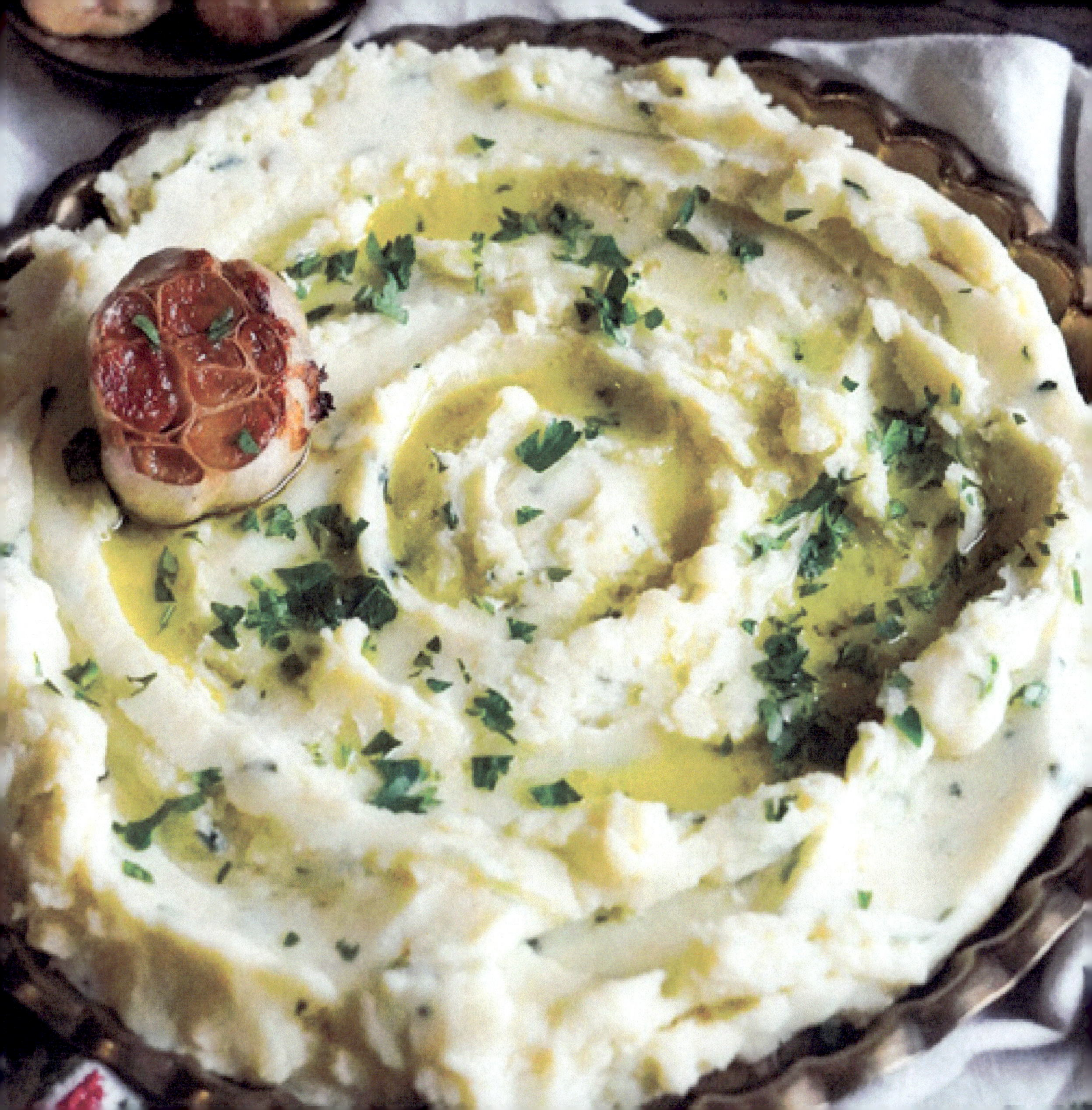

Mutabbal متبل باذنجان

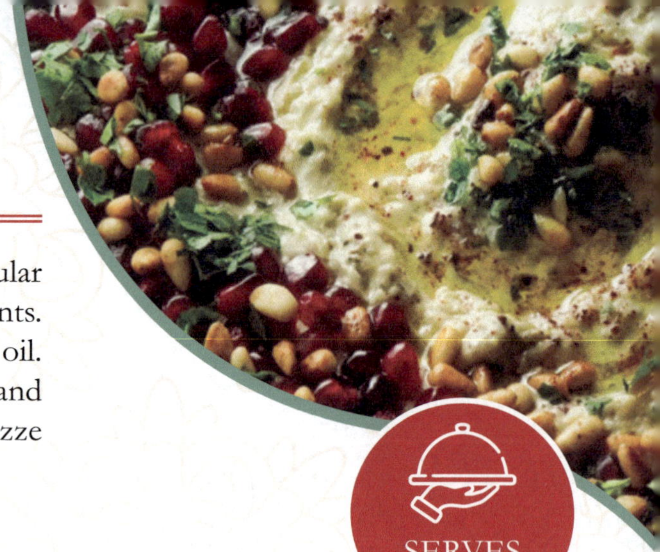

Mutabbal, also mistakenly known as Baba Ganoush, is a popular Middle Eastern dish made from roasted or grilled eggplants. Mutabbal blended with tahini, garlic, lemon juice, and olive oil. Baba Ghanoush doesn' have tahini! Mutabbal is a flavorful and creamy dip or spread that is commonly served as part of mezze (appetizers) in Middle Eastern cuisine.

SERVES 6

INGREDIENTS:

- 2 large eggplants, about 2 pounds
- 6-8 large garlic cloves
- ¼ cup plain whole milk yogurt
- ¼ cup tahini
- 3-4 tablespoons lemon juice (to taste)
- 1 tsp salt, or to taste
- 5 tbsp extra virgin olive oil for brushing
- Toasted pine nuts or almonds

DIRECTIONS:

1. Preheat the oven to 450 degrees F.
2. Cut each eggplant in half lengthwise and place them onto a baking sheet lined with parchment paper.
3. Drizzle each eggplant slice with about 1 tablespoon of olive oil on the flesh side, then flip it to have the flesh face down on the sheet.
4. Place the peeled garlic cloves into a small pocket of foil, and add 1 tablespoon of olive oil on top.
5. Close the aluminum foil pocket and place it into the same tray.
6. Cover and place into the oven for 50 minutes to 1 hour. Remove and let it cool.
7. Peel the skin and scoop the insides into a bowl. Add the yogurt, tahini, salt, roasted garlic, and lemon juice.
8. Mash well, either using a potato masher or a fork.
9. Fry your desired amount of pine nuts or almonds in olive oil for extra flavor.
10. Spoon over ready Mutabbal, making sure to spoon some olive oil as well.

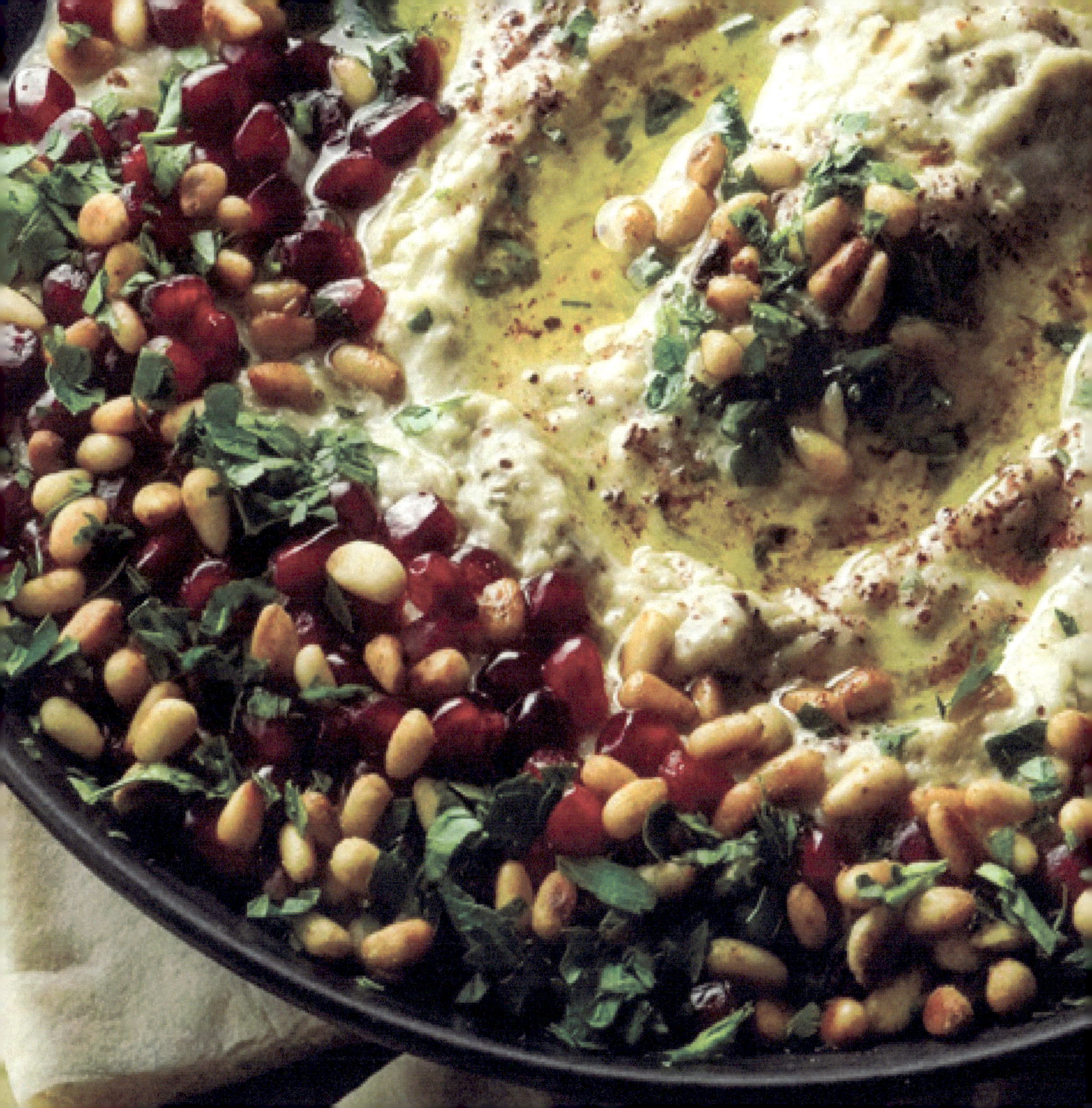

Sahawiq السحاوق اليمنية

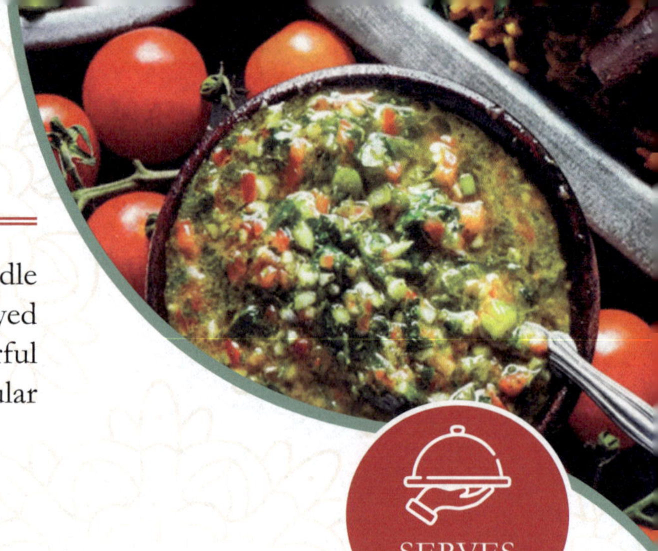

SERVES

Sahawiq, also known as Zhug, is a spicy and aromatic Middle Eastern hot sauce that hails from Yemen and is widely enjoyed across the region. This fiery condiment adds a bold and flavorful kick to various dishes, and its versatile nature makes it a popular addition to Middle Eastern cuisine.

INGREDIENTS:

- 2 large roma tomatoes
- ⅓ cup green onions
- 5 garlic cloves
- 1 jalapeno (or to taste)
- ⅓ cup cilantro
- ½ cup fresh mint
- ¼ of a green bell pepper
- ¼ of a red bell pepper
- ¼ cup extra virgin olive oil
- 1 tsp coriander powder
- ½ tsp cumin
- 1-2 tbsp lemon juice
- Salt to taste

DIRECTIONS:

*Sahawiq is a small salad or salsa, so everything needs to be finely chopped but not watery. In this instance, you can use the food processor and slowly process the vegetables until they're small chunks, or chop by hand.

1. Finely chop the vegetables, preferably by hand, as fine as possible. Combine them in a bowl.
2. Add the lemon juice and olive oil.
3. Finish it off with the cumin, coriander, and your desired amount of salt.

Serve with Zurbian, Mandi, or any rice dish.

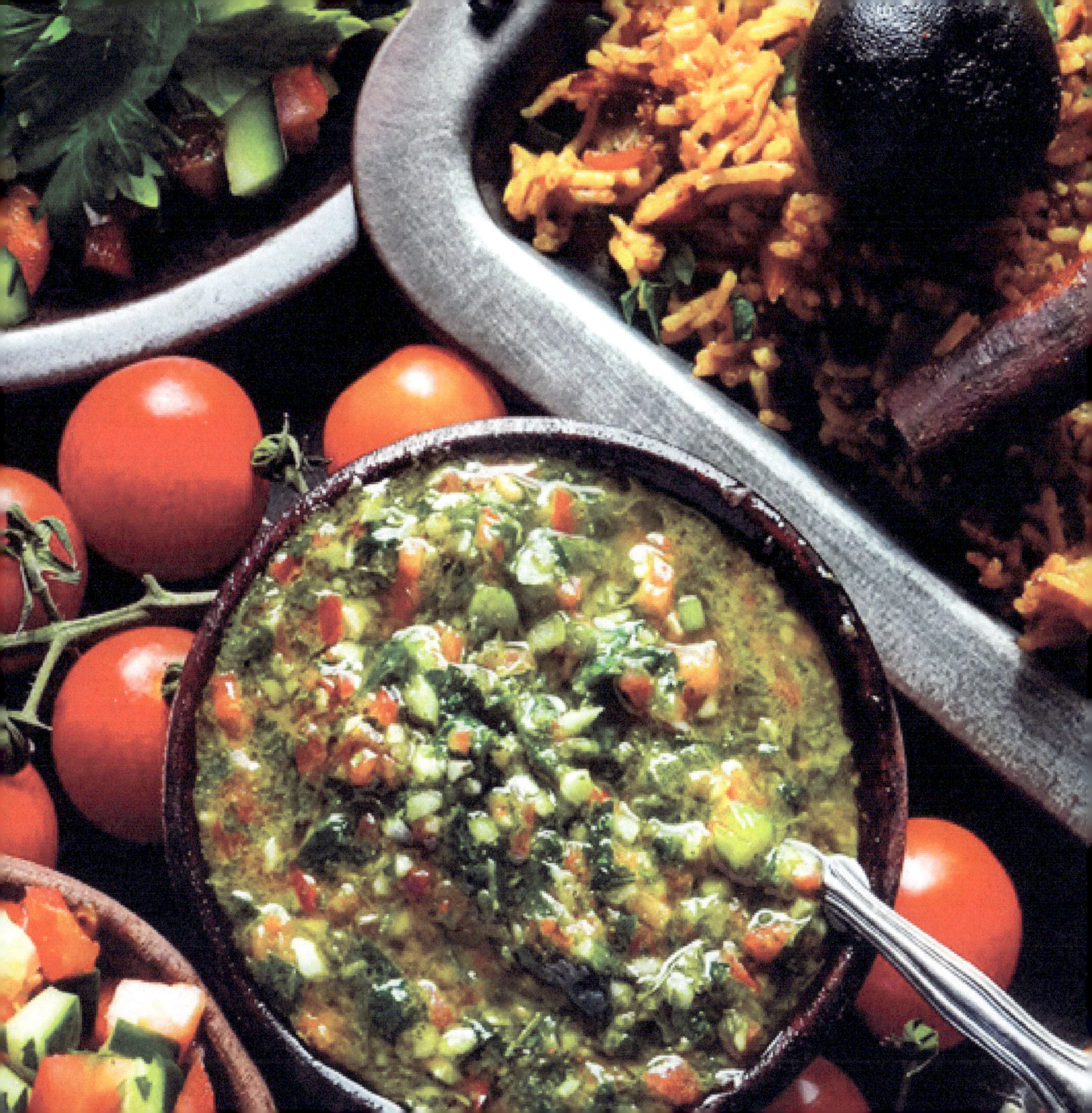

Salatat Mashawi (Mashawi Salad)

سلطة مشاوي

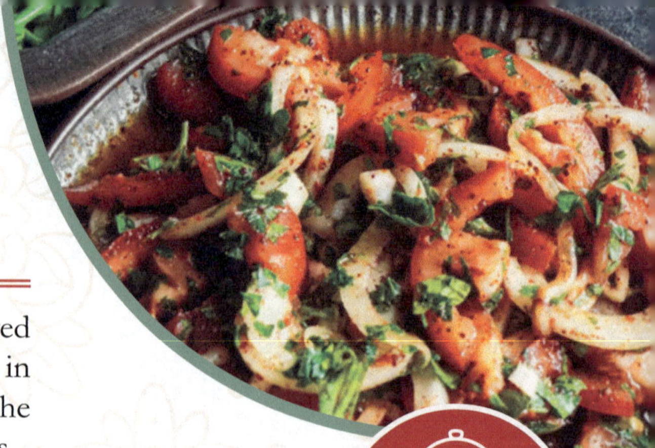

SERVES

"Mashawi Salad" refers to a type of salad commonly served alongside grilled or barbecued meats, known as "mashawi" in Middle Eastern cuisine. The salad is designed to complement the rich flavors of grilled meats with its fresh and vibrant ingredients.

INGREDIENTS:

- ½ a bunch of parsley
- 2 large tomatoes
- 1 medium yellow onion
- 3 tbsp extra virgin olive oil
- 1 tbsp sumac
- Lemon juice, to taste
- Salt, to taste

DIRECTIONS:

1. Slice the tomato and onion into thin strips. Finely chop the parsley leaves.
2. Add the sliced onions, tomatoes, and chopped parsley to a bowl.
3. Add the olive oil, sumac, and add salt and lemon juice to taste.
4. Toss everything well and adjust for extra salt or tang.

Serve next to grilled meats or baked lamb!

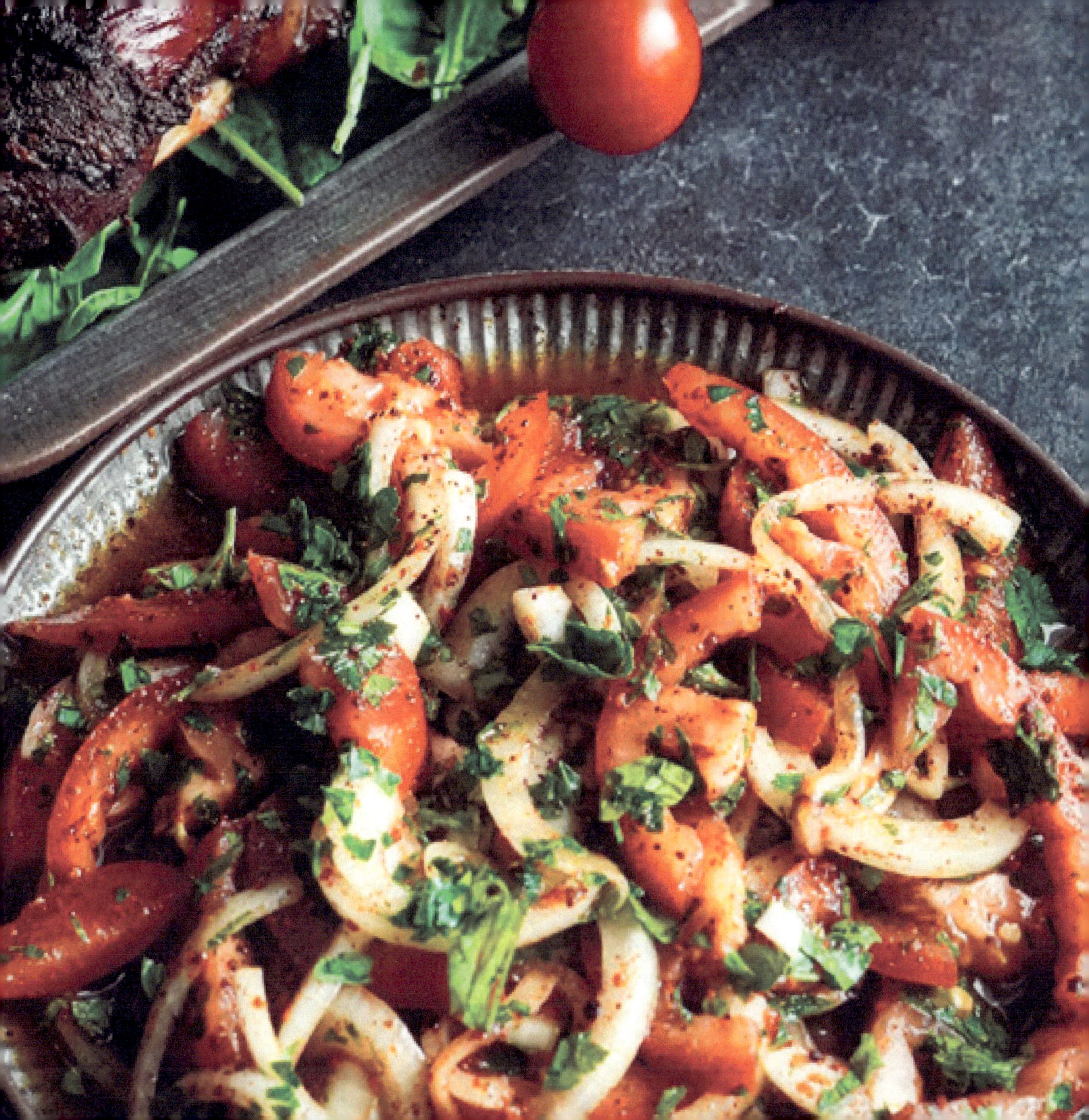

Loubiya Bi Zeit لوبيا بالزيت

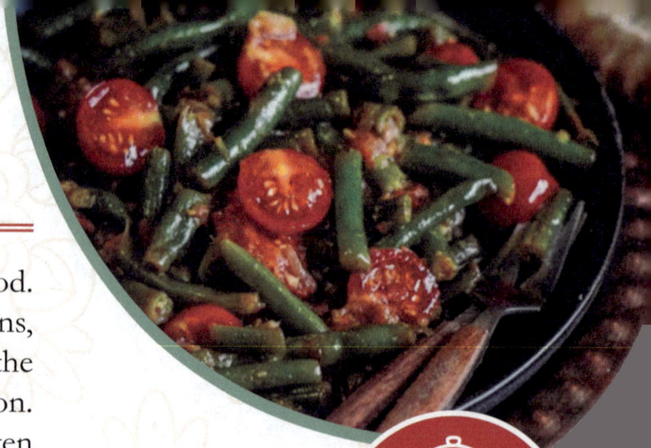

This vegan/vegetarian dish is a classic and delicious comfort food. Tender beans are braised in a mixture of lots of garlic and onions, as well as tomatoes and olive oil. It is most commonly eaten in the summer when tomatoes and green beans are fresh and in season. It's also a meal that can be eaten cold and is refreshing or eaten warm depending on how you like it.

SERVES 3-4

INGREDIENTS:

- 3 cups green beans or long beans (1lb)
- 1 large yellow onion, finely chopped
- 10 garlic cloves, minced
- 3 large tomatoes, cubed small
- 3 tbsp olive oil
- 2 tbsp water
- 1/2 tsp 7 spices
- 1/2 tsp coriander powder
- ¼ tsp of Aleppo pepper
- 1/2 tsp bouillon powder
- 1/4 tsp black pepper
- Salt to taste

DIRECTIONS:

1. Trim the ends off of the beans. Cut the beans into 2-3 inch long pieces.
2. Heat the oil in a medium pot over medium-high heat, add the onions and the garlic. Cook for about 5 minutes or until wilted and golden brown, stirring continuously. Mix in the cut green beans, sprinkle with the bouillon powder, the 7 spices, coriander, Aleppo and black pepper. Reduce heat to moderately low, cover and cook for 15 minutes, stirring occasionally.
3. Add the chopped tomatoes, cover and bring to a boil over medium-high heat. Add in the water and mix. Reduce heat to medium-low and cook for about 15 minutes, or until the beans are tender. Add tomato paste and adjust salt to taste. If the beans need more liquid, add tomato sauce or water, 2 tbsp at a time.
4. Transfer to a serving dish and serve with warm pita bread.

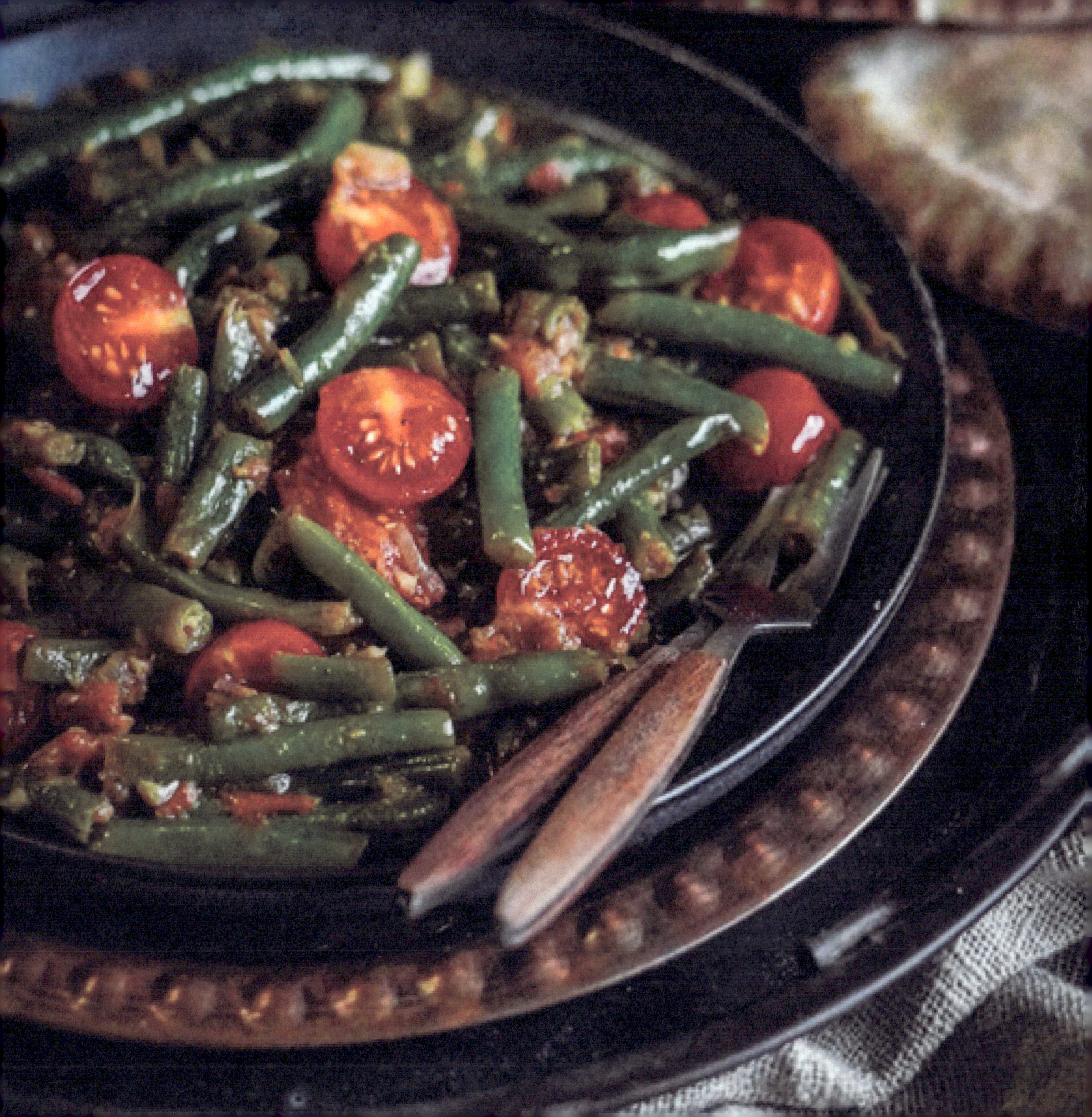

Daqoos (Spicy Garlic Tomato Sauce) دقوس

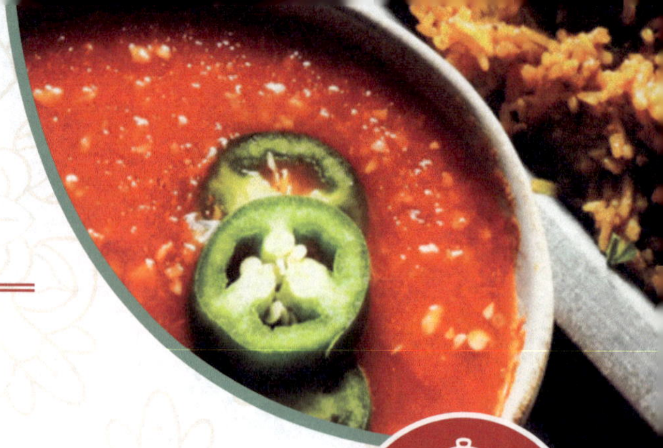

Daqoos is a traditional Middle Eastern sauce that hails from the Arabian Gulf, particularly popular in Kuwait, Saudi Arabia, and other Gulf countries. This savory condiment is a flavorful accompaniment that adds a zesty kick to various dishes.

The base of Daqoos is typically made with ripe tomatoes, garlic, and green chili peppers. These ingredients are finely minced or blended to create a smooth and spicy sauce. The heat from the chili peppers provides a distinct kick, while garlic adds depth and flavor. Some variations may include additional spices like cumin or coriander for extra aromatic complexity.

SERVES

INGREDIENTS:

- 2 tbsp extra virgin olive oil
- 5 garlic cloves, minced
- 1 jalapeno, or to taste
- 15 oz tomato sauce
- 1 cup water
- ½ tsp garlic powder
- 1 tsp salt
- ¼ tsp black pepper

DIRECTIONS:

1. To start, begin by heating up 2 tablespoons of extra virgin olive oil in a pot on medium-high heat.
2. Add in the minced garlic and jalapeno. You can leave the jalapeno seeds in for extra heat. I prefer chopping the jalapeno into circles to easily remove them or identify them when serving.
3. Saute the garlic and jalapeno until the garlic turns a golden color.
4. Add the tomato sauce, and the water.
5. Stir in the salt, garlic powder, and black pepper. Cover and let this simmer for 3 minutes on medium-low, or until thickened.
6. Serve with kabsa, fish, or any main dish.

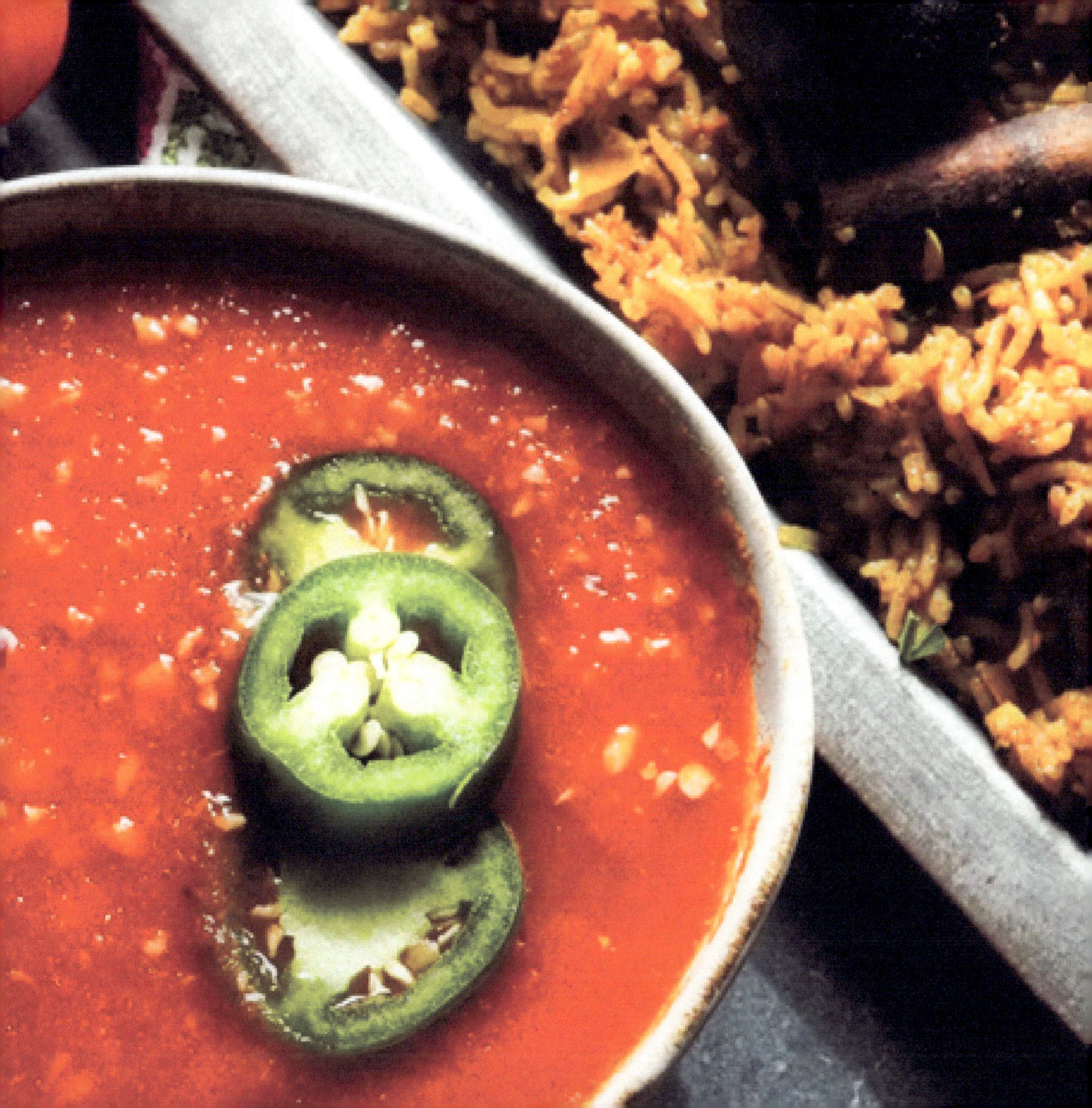

Sumac Onion Salad سلطة البصل والسماق

Sumac Onion Salad is a refreshing and tangy salad that highlights the citrusy and slightly tart flavor of sumac. Sumac, a deep red spice derived from the berries of the sumac shrub, adds a unique and vibrant element to the salad. It's commonly used in salads and other Middle Eastern dishes. This salad is the perfect accompaniment next to chicken or lamb.

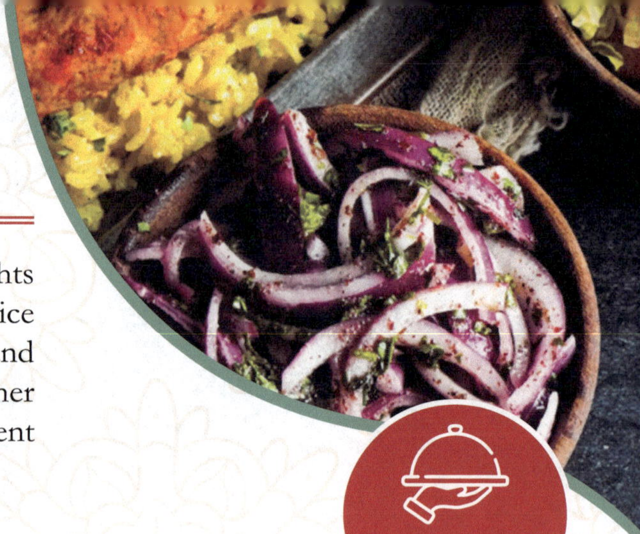

SERVES

INGREDIENTS:

- 1 large red onion, sliced into thin wings
- 1 tbsp sumac
- 1 tbsp extra virgin olive oil
- 3 tbsp parsley, finely chopped
- Salt, to taste

DIRECTIONS:

1. Combine all the ingredients in a bowl and toss them together.
2. Taste for seasoning and adjust as needed. For example, if you feel it needs more salt, or sumac. If you're not using good quality sumac, you might need to add some lemon juice for tang.
3. Let marinate while you complete your cooking or eat right away.

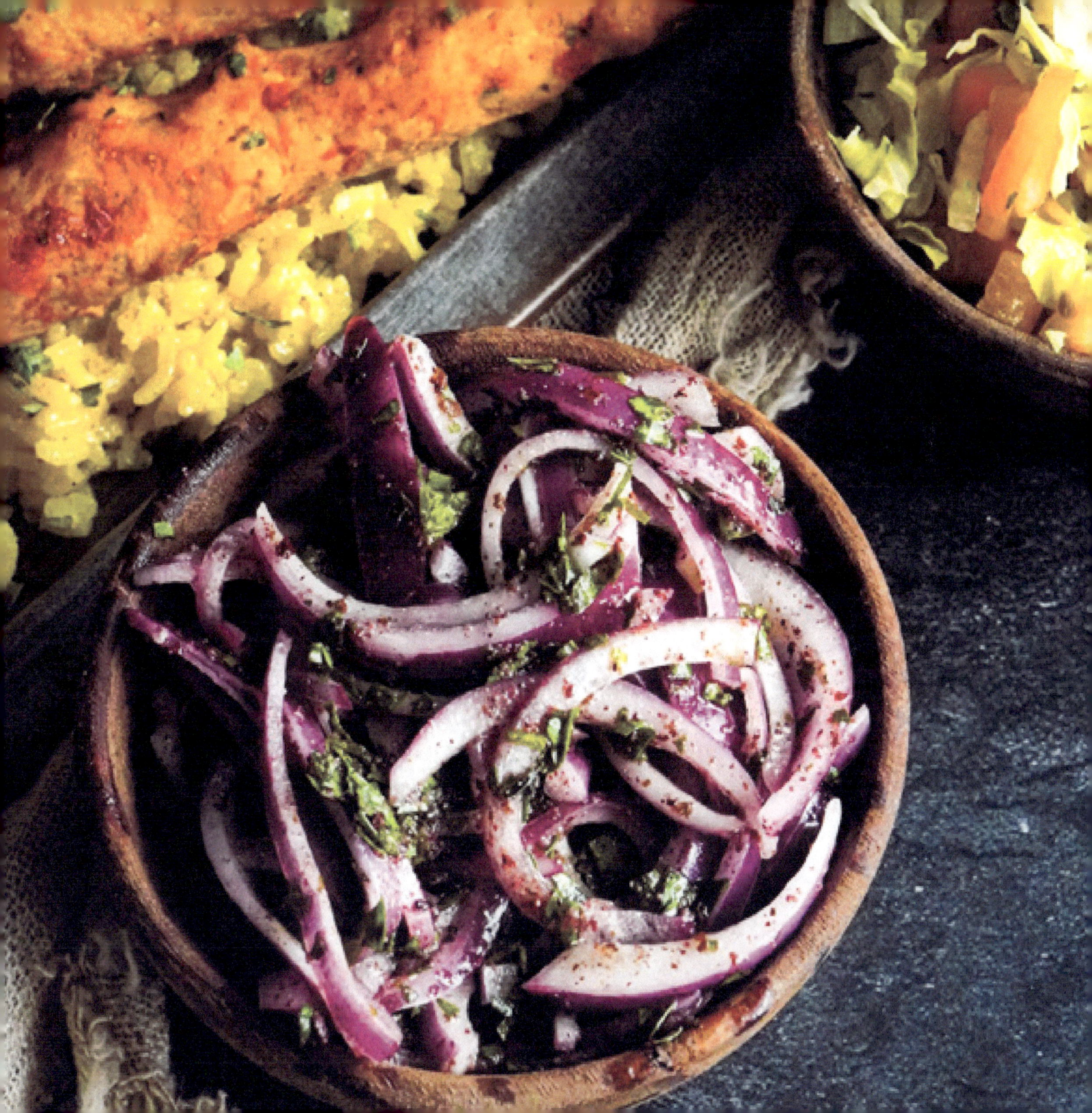

Salata Arabiya سلطة عربية

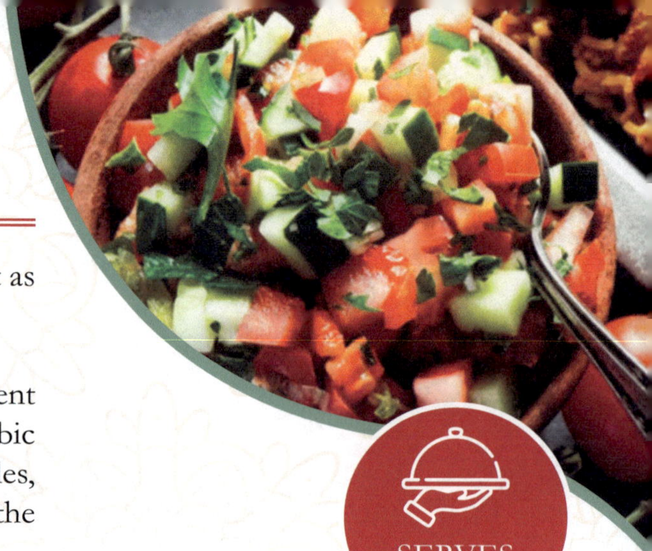

This is a traditional Middle Eastern salad that many prefer to eat as a side dish.

These days, people are familiar with many kinds of different salads. One of the easiest, yet flavorful, ones to make is this Arabic Chopped Salad. All you need to do is get some fresh vegetables, wash them thoroughly, chop, and you're ready to serve. It is the perfect side salad during Ramadan!

SERVES

INGREDIENTS:

Salad:

- 2 large tomatoes
- 3 large radishes
- 1 romaine heart
- ⅓ of a green onion
- ¼ cup parsley
- ½ large cucumber or 3 small Persian Cucumbers

Dressing:

- 1 tsp sumac
- 1 lemon's juice
- ½ teaspoon salt
- 3 tbsp olive oil

DIRECTIONS:

1. Chop all the vegetables finely.
2. Mix the dressing ingredients together and pour over your chopped vegetables.

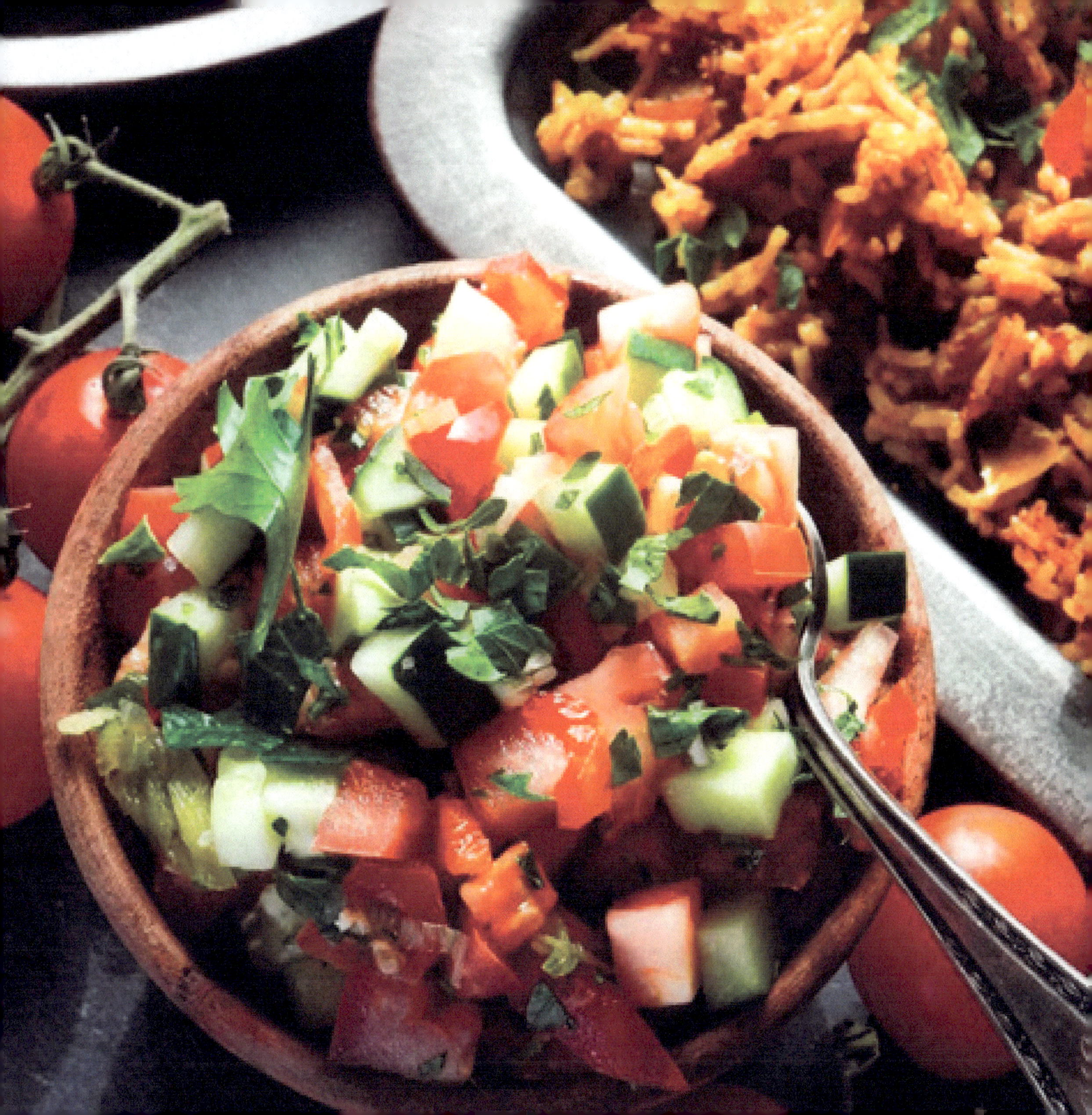

Lentil and Swiss Chard Soup شوربة العدس بالسلق

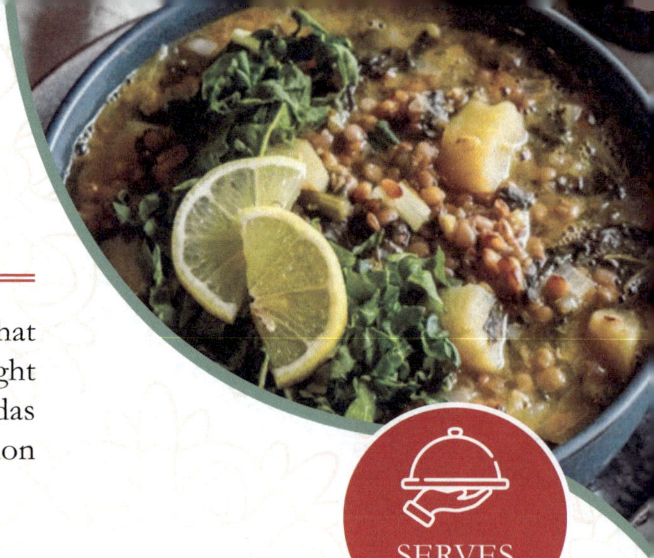

Lentil Swiss Chard Soup is a hearty and nutritious soup that combines the earthy flavors of lentils with the vibrant and light taste of Swiss chard. More often than not, it is referred to as "Adas Bi Hamid" meaning lentils with lemon for the use of fresh lemon juice in the soup.

SERVES 4

INGREDIENTS:

- 3 tbsp extra virgin olive oil
- 1 large yellow onion, finely chopped
- 3 garlic cloves, minced
- 1 cup green lentils, washed
- 3 small potatoes, peeled and cubed
- 3 cups chopped swiss chard, about 1 bunch
- 6½ cups hot water
- ¾ tsp coriander powder
- Salt, to taste
- ½ tsp black pepper
- 3 tbsp freshly squeezed lemon juice, or to taste

DIRECTIONS:

1. Add a pot to the stove to medium-high heat.
2. Add the olive oil and heat up for a minute before adding in the finely chopped onion and the garlic. Saute until translucent, about 5 minutes or so.
3. Add the cubed potatoes and mix.
4. Wash and drain the lentils and add them to the pot.
5. Add the water to cover and let it cook covered for about 15 minutes, or until the potatoes and lentils are cooked and softened.
6. Wash and chop the swiss chard.
7. Add to the pot, along with the salt and black pepper. Stir.
8. Cover and let it simmer for another 10 minutes
9. Stir in the lemon juice and serve

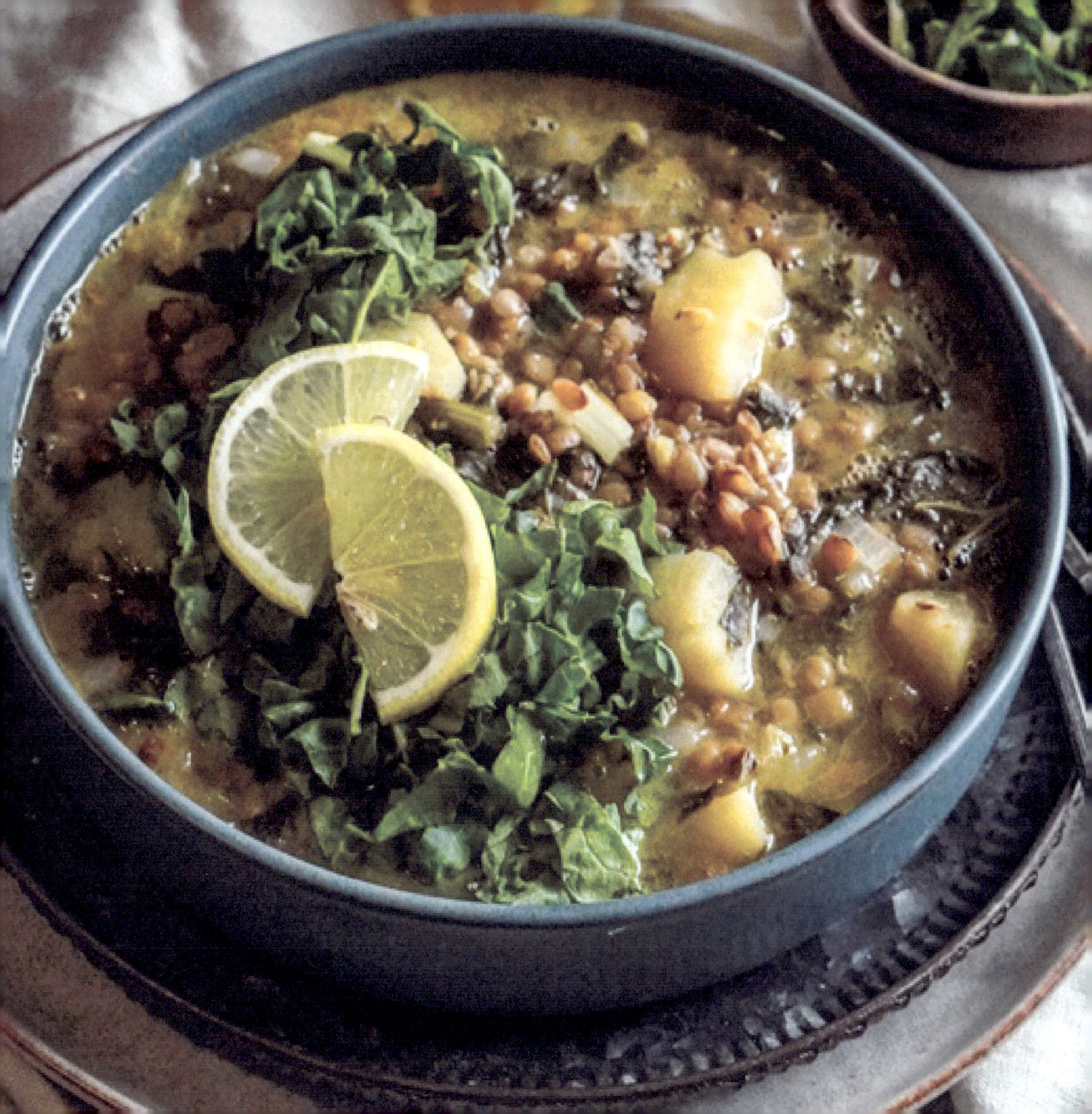

Cauliflower Yogurt Salad

سلطة القرنبيط

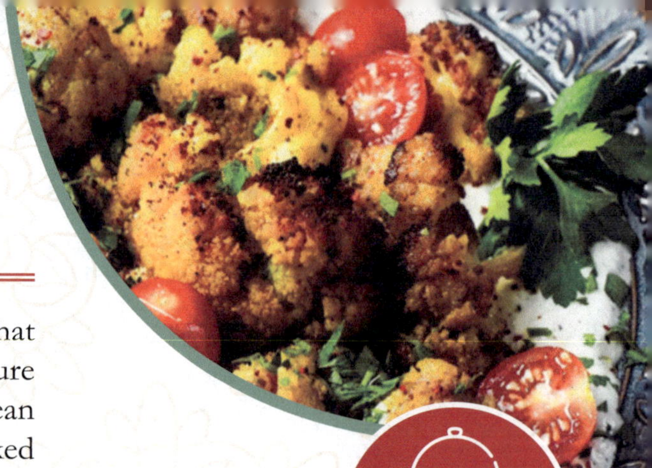

Cauliflower yogurt salad is a refreshing and nutritious dish that combines the subtle flavor of cauliflower with the creamy texture of yogurt. It's a popular salad in Middle Eastern and Mediterranean cuisines, often enjoyed as a side dish or a light appetizer. It's packed full of flavor and it's easy to put together.

SERVES

INGREDIENTS:

- 1 large head of cauliflower, 2-2½ lbs
- ¼ cup extra virgin olive oil
- 1 tsp salt
- 1 tsp paprika
- ½ tsp turmeric
- 1 tsp garlic powder
- 1 tsp 7 spices
- ½ tsp Aleppo pepper

Yogurt Sauce:

- 1 ½ cups plain whole milk yogurt
- 1 tsp sumac
- ½ tsp Aleppo pepper
- Lemon juice, to taste
- Salt, to taste

To Serve:

- Chopped tomatoes
- Chopped parsley
- Toasted pine nuts, optional
- Pomegranate seeds, optional

DIRECTIONS:

1. Preheat the oven to 425 F.
2. Prepare a baking sheet and line it with parchment paper.
3. Cut the cauliflower into single florets, about 1 ½ inches in size.
4. Mix the extra virgin olive oil with the salt, paprika, turmeric, garlic powder, 7 spices, and Aleppo pepper.
5. Spread the cauliflower florets onto the prepared baking sheet.
6. Drizzle the olive oil and spices mixture on top, and toss by hand to coat the cauliflower evenly.

7. Bake at 425 F for 20-25 minutes, or until tender and golden. Set aside.
8. To make the yogurt sauce, combine the yogurt, sumac, and Aleppo pepper in a bowl. Add salt and lemon juice to taste.
9. To serve, spread the yogurt onto the bottom of a serving plate or platter.
10. Top with the cooked cauliflower.
11. Garnish with chopped tomatoes, chopped parsley, and pine nuts and pomegranates if desired.

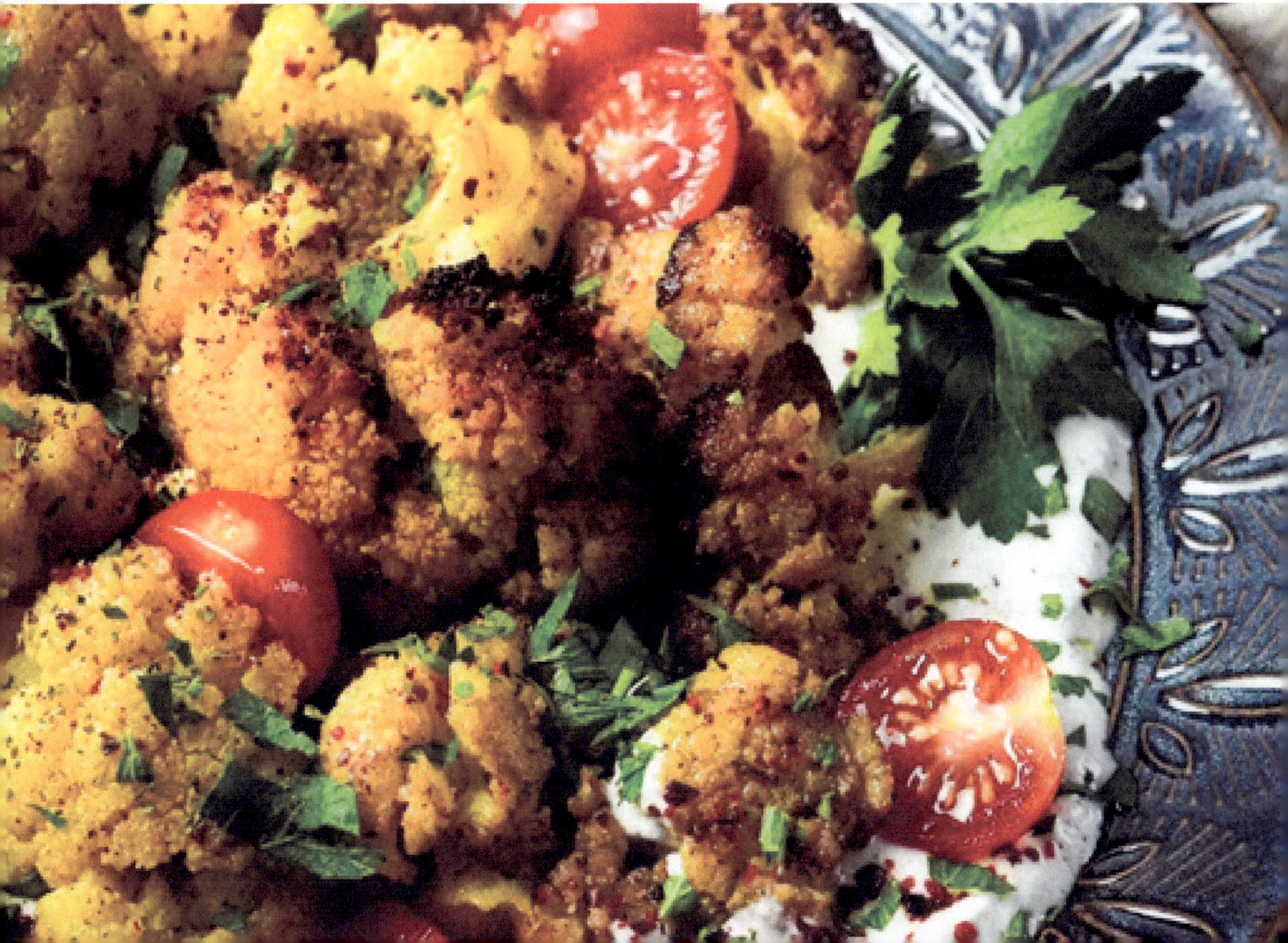

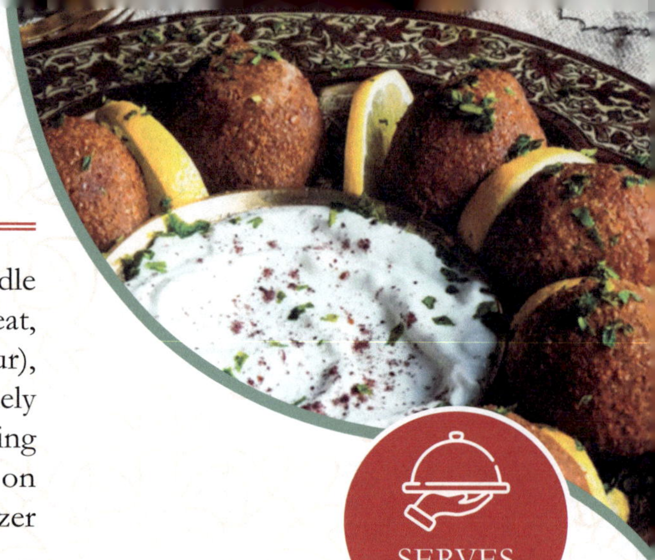

Kubbeh كبة

Kubbeh, also spelled kibbeh or kubba, is a traditional Middle Eastern dish that showcases the artistry of combining ground meat, typically lamb or beef, with cracked wheat (burghul or bulgur), onions, and an array of aromatic spices. The mixture is finely ground and shaped into distinctive oval or round forms, creating a versatile base for various preparations.These are always found on Ramadan iftar tables too, and this recipe makes the perfect freezer batch.

SERVES

INGREDIENTS:

For The Outer Shell:

- 3¼ cups fine burghul (bulgur wheat)
- 4 cups boiling water
- ¼ cup red onion
- 1 tsp aleppo pepper
- ½ tsp cumin
- 1½ tsp salt
- 1 tsp paprika
- 1 lb lean ground beef, 93% lean or more
- 8 tbsp cold water

For The Filling:

- 1 lb ground beef, 80% lean
- 1 tbsp oil, any
- 1 tbsp ghee
- 1 medium yellow onion, finely chopped
- 1½ tsp 7 spices
- ¼ tsp cumin
- 1 tsp pomegranate molasses
- ½ tsp cinnamon
- 1½ tsp salt
- ¼ tsp black pepper
- 1 tsp paprika
- 1 tsp sumac
- Fried pine nuts

DIRECTIONS:

To Make Kubbeh Dough

1. Add the burghul to a large bowl, then pour the boiling water on top.
2. Cover the bowl, and let it sit for 30-45 minutes.

3. While it's still hot or warm, mix the burghul well with your hands, kneading the dough between your fingers and clumping it together so the burghul gets finer.
4. An optional step is to add the burghul to a food processor and pulse until fine before adding the water.
5. Once kneaded, add the super finely chopped onion(preferably chopped in a food processor), Aleppo pepper, cumin, paprika, and salt to the kubbeh dough. Then, add the lean beef and mix well.
6. Add cold water to get the smooth and emulsified consistency, then cover and allow it to cool in the fridge until completely cold. .

To Make The Filling

1. Add the oil and ghee to a skillet on medium-high heat. Then, add the beef and sauté until the liquid has almost evaporated.
2. Add the finely chopped onion, 7 spices, cumin, cinnamon, salt, black pepper, paprika, sumac, and pomegranate molasses to the pan. Cook all the way through.
3. Add fried nuts to taste and let it cool before filling the kubbeh.

To Form And Fry Kubbeh Balls

1. Grab a ping pong size ball of the cooled bulgur mix and start shaping it by poking it through the middle and almost coring it with your finger to make a deep hole or football shape.
2. Stuff it with the ground beef mixture and close the other end. If the mix keeps cracking, keep the bowl of cold water mixed and cornstarch on hand. Use it sparingly by adding a few drops to your fingers when needing to fix a crack. Once shaped, lay on a baking sheet lined with parchment paper to air dry.
3. You can immediately deep fry the kubbeh in hot oil that's been previously heated on medium high heat until they become golden brown.
4. You could also save them for the freezer. Keep them on the baking sheet lined with parchment paper, and wrap with plastic wrap. Freeze until completely frozen, then you can transfer to ziplock bags with the amounts of your choosing and freeze again.

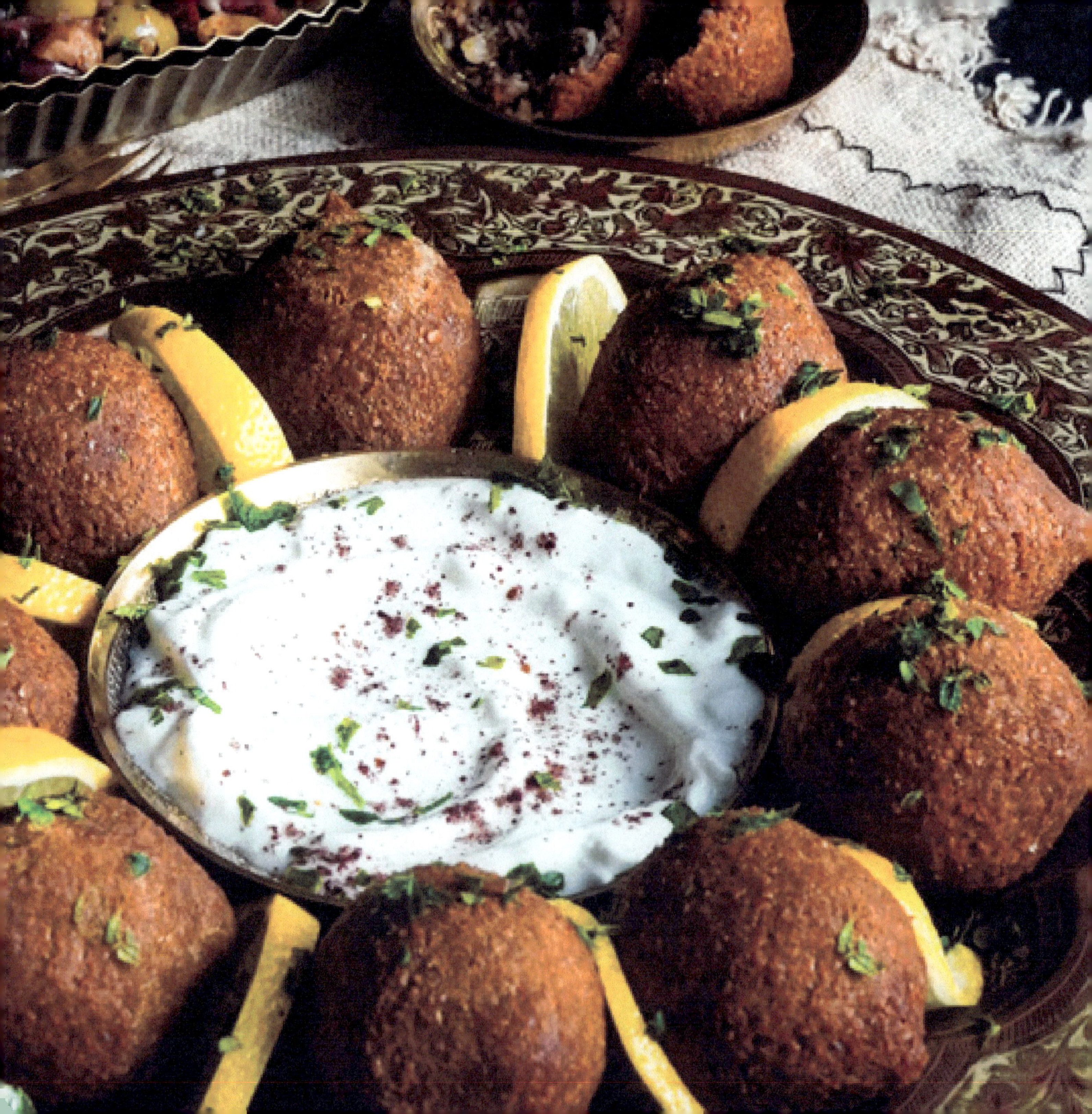

Arab Mains & Entrees

أطباق رئيسية

The enchanting world of Arab cuisine is where every bite is a celebration of centuries-old culinary traditions, a true testament to the region's rich history, and an invitation to savor flavor. Arab entrees are a kaleidoscope of tastes and textures, reflecting the diversity of the Arab world, from the shores of the Mediterranean to the Arabian Peninsula.

Arab entrees are a symphony of spices, herbs, and carefully selected ingredients that come together to create a culinary experience unlike any other. Whether it's the aromatic embrace of slow-cooked stews, the enticing fragrance of grilled meats, or the delicate balance of rice and savory accompaniments, Arab entrees are a journey through a landscape of flavorful delights.

The following Middle Eastern main dishes represent not just a culmination of flavors but a celebration of cultural identity and centuries of culinary innovation.

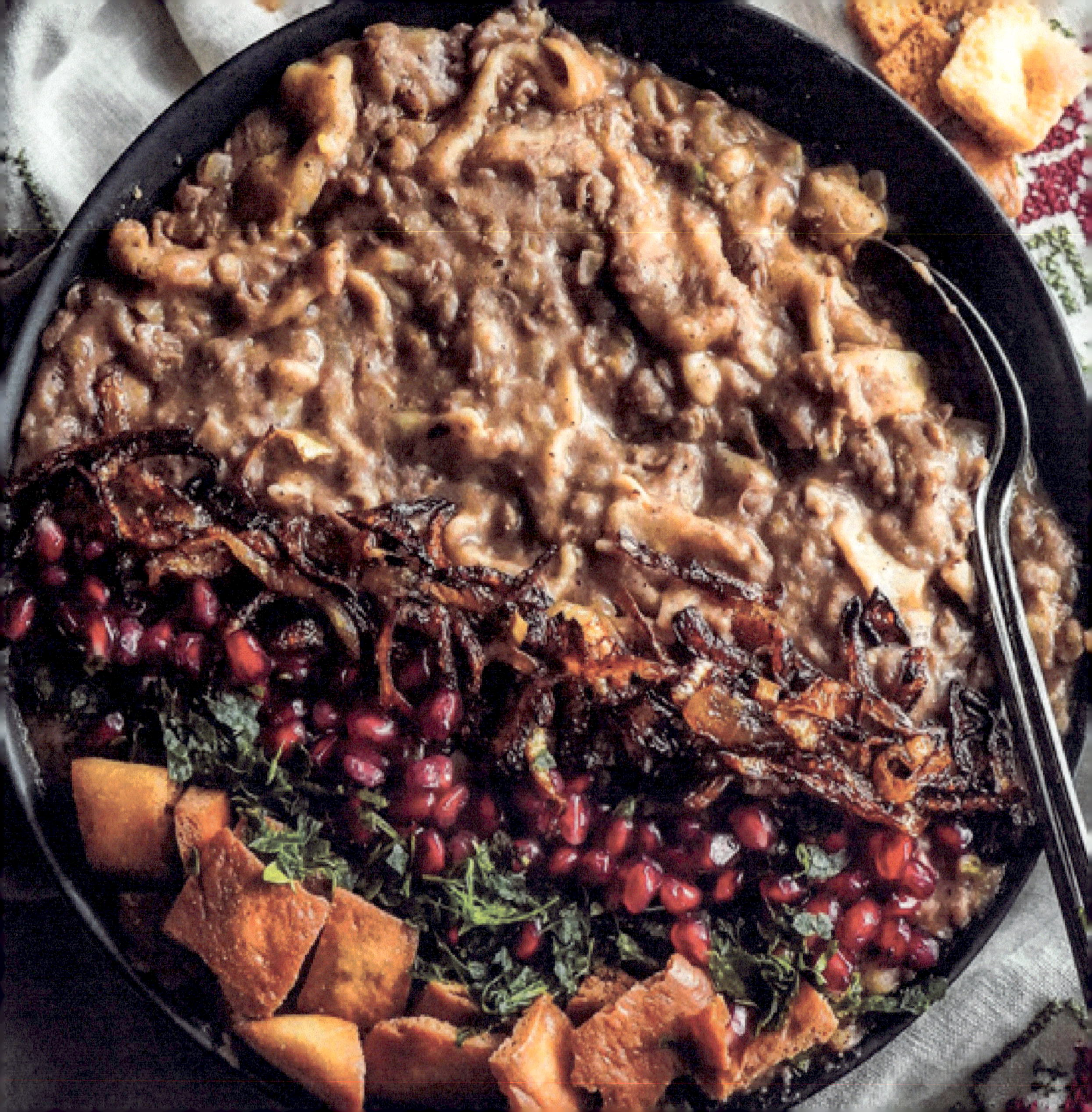

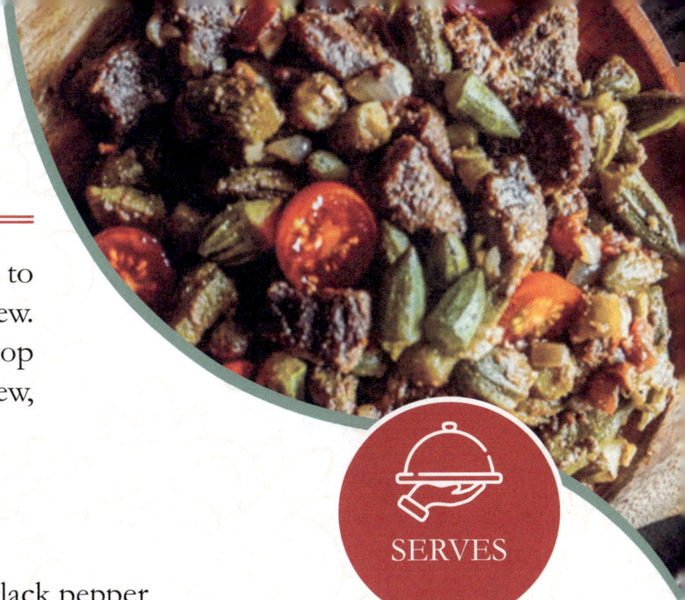

Bamiya Bil Saniyeh بامية بالصينية

Bamiya Bil Saniyeh translates to "Okra in a pan" in reference to making it differently than the typical okra (Bamiya) tomato stew. This bamiya is baked, and is easier to prepare than the stovetop version. It utilizes nearly identical ingredients as the bamiya stew, but with less preparation work.

SERVES

INGREDIENTS:

- 1 lb beef stew meat, cut into 1 inch cubes
- 1 14 oz bag of frozen okra (bamiya)
- 1 large yellow onion
- 1 large tomato
- 5 garlic cloves
- 1 teaspoon salt
- 2 tsp7 spices
- 1 tsp garlic powder
- 1 tsp onion powder
- ½ tsp paprika
- ½ tsp black pepper
- ¼ cup extra virgin olive oil
- 1 ½ tbsp white vinegar
- 2 tbsp water

Pro Tip: If you want the beef to be more tender and to cook quicker, use a great cut of beef like sirloin or tenderloin. Middle Eastern stews and bakes typically use stew meat to cut costs while maintaining an integral part of a dish.

DIRECTIONS:

1. Preheat your oven to 350 F.
2. I like to begin by washing (soaking) the beef before using it in a mixture of water, vinegar, and salt. I find that this gets rid of any excess blood that remains on the beef, along with any residual smells. Once done, I give it an extra rinse and pat it dry. You could completely forgo this step.
3. Prepare a 9x13 pan with parchment paper, and add the cubed beef.
4. Add the finely chopped onion, minced garlic, and chopped tomato.
5. Add the baby okra, both thawed and frozen are okay here, and sprinkle the seasonings on top.

6. Add the water, extra virgin olive oil, and vinegar. Mix everything together well, making sure everything is well spread out and seasoned.
7. Cover the pan with aluminum foil and bake at 350 F for 40 minutes, or until the beef is tender.

Serve with warm pita bread and Arabic salad.

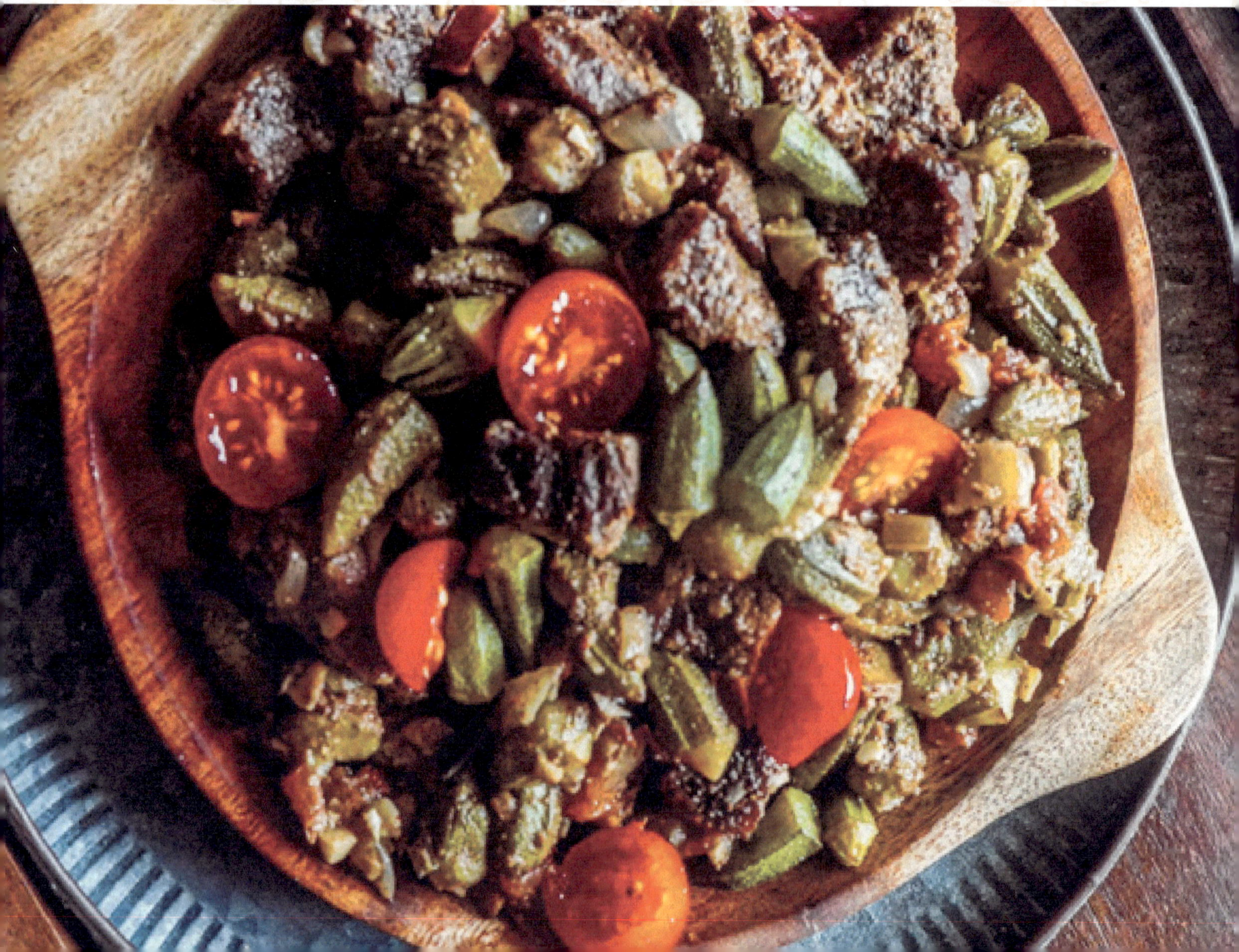

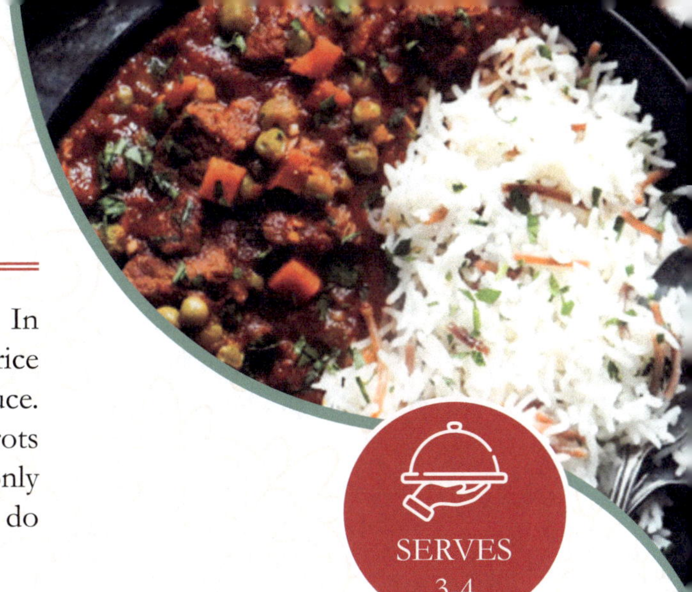

Bazella Ou Jazar (Peas & Carrots Beef Stew) يخنة بازيلا وجزر

Stews, in Arabic, are often referred to as Yakhneh or Tabeekh. In most cases, stews in the Arab world are often accompanied by rice and meat, and some type of vegetable in a tomato or yogurt sauce. Most often they are topped with fried garlic. This peas and carrots stew is a childhood comfort food for many, and it is commonly loved by children. I love this dish, however simple it is, and so do my toddlers. It's easy, delicious, and comforting.

SERVES 3-4

INGREDIENTS:

- 1 packet frozen peas and carrots (16 oz, 454g)
- 1 lb sirloin, cubed (454g)
- 1 tsp garlic powder
- 1 tsp onion powder
- 1 tsp 7 spices
- ½ tsp black pepper
- ¼ tsp cinnamon
- 1 tsp coriander powder
- 3 tbsp olive oil
- 1 medium yellow onion, finely diced
- 15 oz tomato sauce, 1 can (425g)
- 1 tbsp tomato paste
- 3 cups water
- 1 tsp bouillon powder
- Salt to taste

Tassha(Garlic topping):

- 8 cloves garlic, minced
- 1 tbsp oil or butter

DIRECTIONS:

1. To begin, heat up the olive oil on high heat. Add the finely chopped onion and saute until translucent, about 3 minutes.
2. Add the cubed beef and saute until browned, about 8-10 minutes on high heat. Add the 7 spices, garlic powder, onion powder, cinnamon, black pepper, coriander powder, and bouillon powder. Mix well. Add the hot water and mix well. Let it come to a boil for 3-5 minutes before reducing the heat to low, and letting the beef simmer for about 30-40 minutes, until tender.

3. Once tender, remove 1 cup of broth from the pot and dissolve the tomato paste in it. Return it back to the pot along with the tomato sauce.
4. Add the packet of frozen peas and carrots, and mix. Close the lid and let it cook for 15 minutes, until the vegetables are softened. Adjust for salt.
5. In a separate pan, heat 1 tbsp of oil on high heat. Add the minced garlic and saute until golden brown. Add the garlic and the oil on top of the peas and carrots stew. Mix well.
6. Serve with vermicelli rice and lemon wedges.

Pro Tip: If the sauce is too liquidy, let it simmer for another 10-15 minutes to thicken. It will also thicken the more it sits. If the sauce is too thick, add some hot water and adjust the salt to achieve desired thickness and taste.

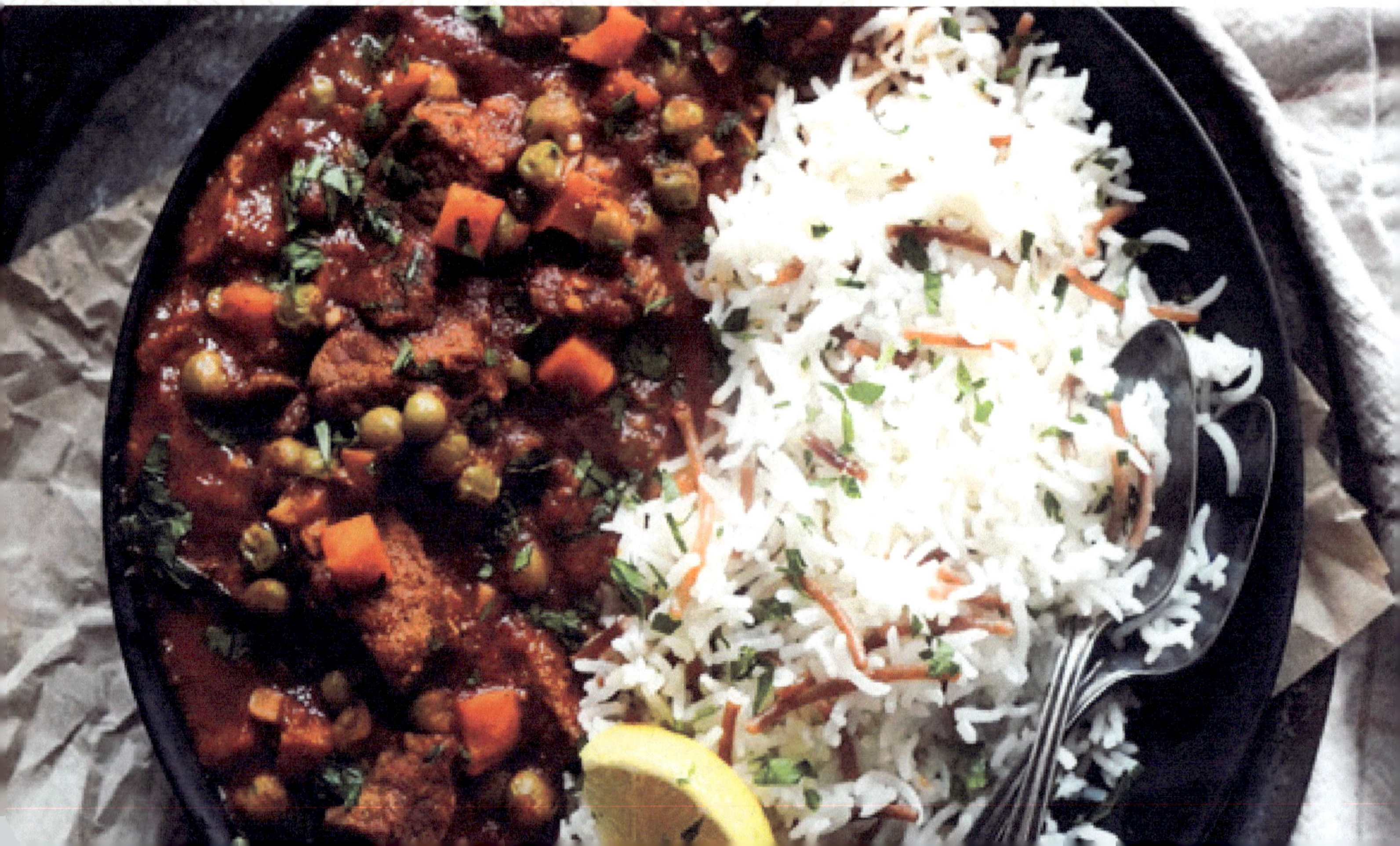

Beitenjan Mahshi (Stuffed Eggplant) باذنجان محشي

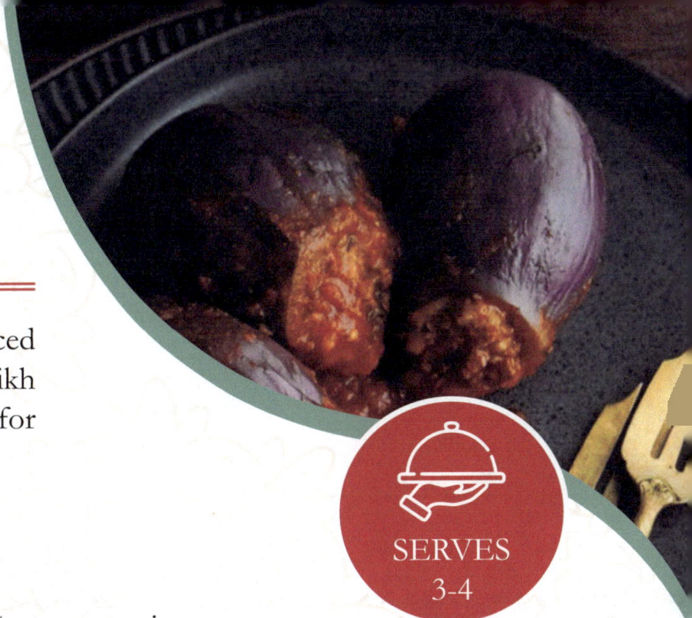

SERVES
3-4

Beitenjan Mahshi is a fried eggplant stuffed with a delicious spiced rice and ground beef filling. It is commonly referred to as "Sheikh Al Mahshi" which translates to"The King of Stuffed Dishes" for its alluring taste and simplicity.

INGREDIENTS:

- 8 baby eggplants
- ½ cup short grain rice, washed and soaked
- ½ pound 80/20 lean ground beef (226g)
- 1 medium roma tomato, chopped small
- 4 garlic cloves, minced
- ¼ cup parsley, finely chopped
- ¼ tsp 7 spices
- ½ tsp coriander powder
- 1 tsp salt
- ¼ tsp turmeric
- ½ tsp black pepper

Tomato Sauce:

- 2 15 oz cans tomato sauce (850g)
- 15 oz water (850g) (measured in the tomato sauce can)
- ½ tsp salt
- 2 tsp extra virgin olive oil

DIRECTIONS:

1. To start, cut the stem off the eggplants, and core them. You'll want to core them carefully so as to not pierce the walls.
2. Once all the eggplants are cored, add them to a large bowl and cover with water, and 1 tbsp of salt. Let them soak for 20 minutes to remove the bitterness. Once soaked, rinse and pat dry.
3. Now, shallow fry the eggplant on all sides and set aside. You could also skip the frying all together.
4. In the meantime, wash and soak the rice. Discard the excess water.
5. Finely chop the parsley, tomato, and garlic. Alternatively, add them to a food process until fine but not liquidy.

6. Add the soaked and drained rice into a large bowl. Add the ground beef, along with the turmeric, black pepper, coriander powder, 7 spices, and salt. Add the vegetable mixture and mix well.
7. Add the filling into the eggplants, leaving about ¼ inch of room at the top of the eggplant. Lay the eggplant in the bottom of a pot, making sure to stack them well.
8. To make the sauce, mix together the tomato sauce, water, olive oil, and salt. Mix well and pour over the eggplants.
9. Cook on high heat for 5 minutes, before reducing the heat to medium-low and simmering for 20-30 minutes, or until the rice is cooked, and the meat is cooked all the way through.
10. Serve with extra sauce to dip the eggplant in and enjoy.

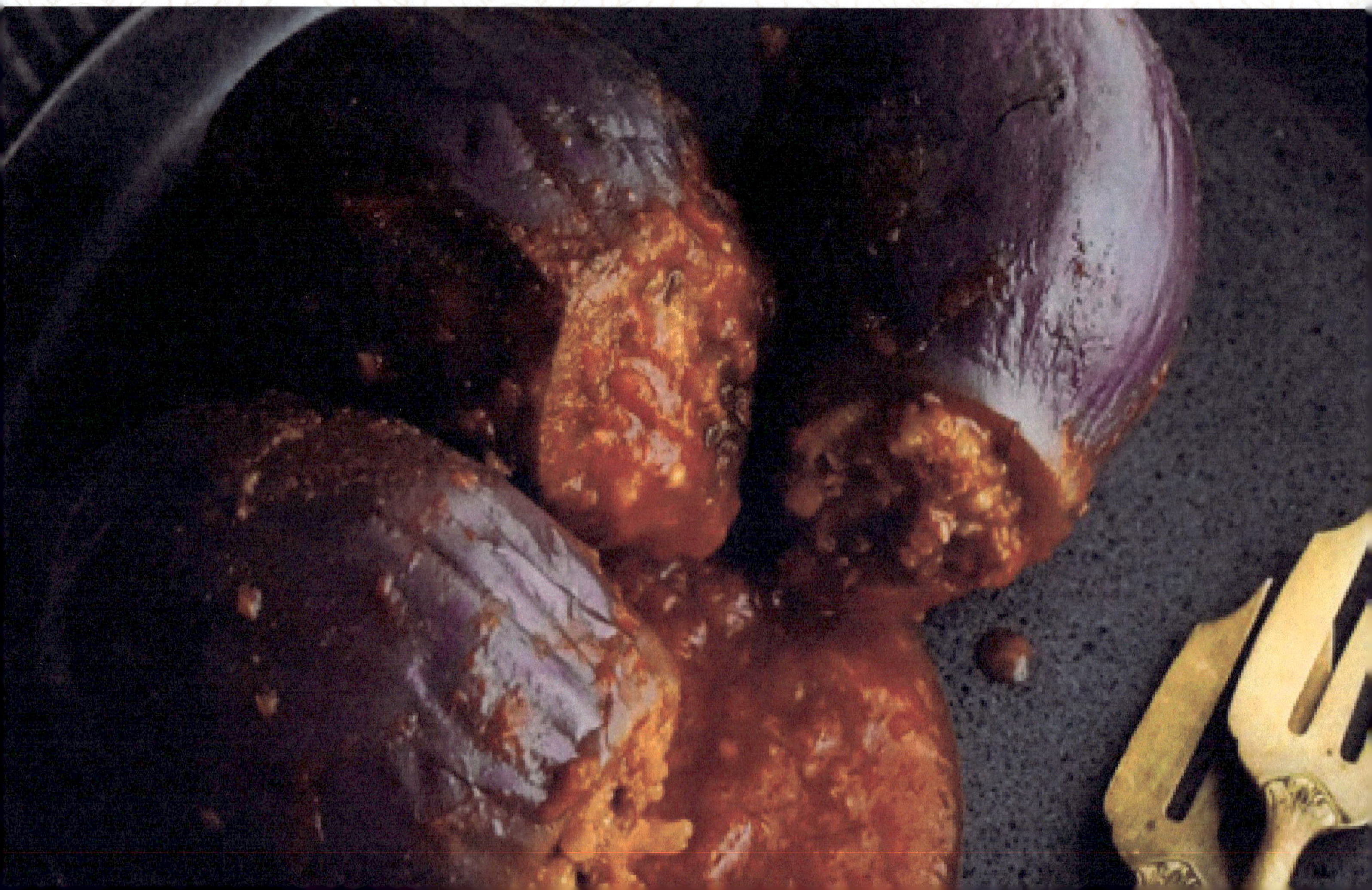

Chicken Shish Tawook Wraps

سندويشات شيش طاووق

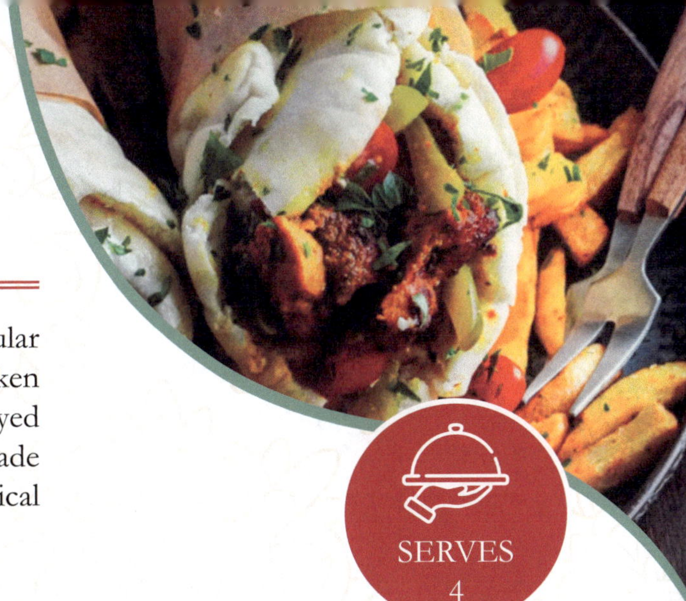

SERVES 4

Chicken Shish Tawook, also known as Shish Taouk, is a popular Middle Eastern dish known for its grilled marinated chicken skewers. It's a flavorful and aromatic dish that is widely enjoyed across the region. These wraps are flavor bomb perfection, made with tender shish tawook pieces and accompanied by the typical Arab sandwich and wrap pairings.

INGREDIENTS:

- 2 lbs chicken breast, cut into cubes
- 4 garlic cloves
- ½ a red bell pepper
- 1 roma tomato
- ¼ cup parsley
- ¼ cup green onions
- 2 tbsp red pepper paste
- 2 tbsp extra virgin olive oil
- Juice of ½ a lemon
- 1 tbsp pomegranate molasses
- 2 tbsp plain whole milk yogurt

Spices:

- 1 tsp garlic powder
- 1 tsp onion powder
- 1 ½ tsp 7 spices
- 1 ½ tsp coriander powder
- 1 tsp Aleppo pepper
- 1 ½ tsp salt, or to taste
- 1 tsp paprika
- ¾ tsp sumac

To Serve:

- Pita bread
- Garlic sauce
- French fries
- Middle Eastern pickled cucumbers
- Tomatoes
- Lettuce

DIRECTIONS:

1. Begin by cutting the chicken breast into 1½ -2 inch cubes. Transfer to a large bowl.
2. Add the tomato, parsley, garlic, green onions, and bell pepper to a food processor. Process but keep it chunky.
3. Add the processed vegetables to the chicken.
4. Now, add in the pepper paste, the yogurt, pomegranate molasses, lemon juice, and olive oil. Give everything a good mix. Add all the seasonings and make sure each chicken piece is well coated. Cover and let it marinate for a minimum of 3 hours, preferably overnight.
5. Remove the chicken from the marinade and place in a single layer in the air fryer basket. Set the air fryer to 370°F and cook the chicken for 10 minutes.
6. Open the air fryer and flip over the chicken. Set the air fryer to 370°F and cook the chicken for another 5 minutes.
7. Test with a meat thermometer to ensure the chicken has reached an internal temperature of 165°F.
8. To serve, spread some garlic sauce on pita bread. Add a few cooked chicken pieces. Add some french fries, pickles, and vegetables.

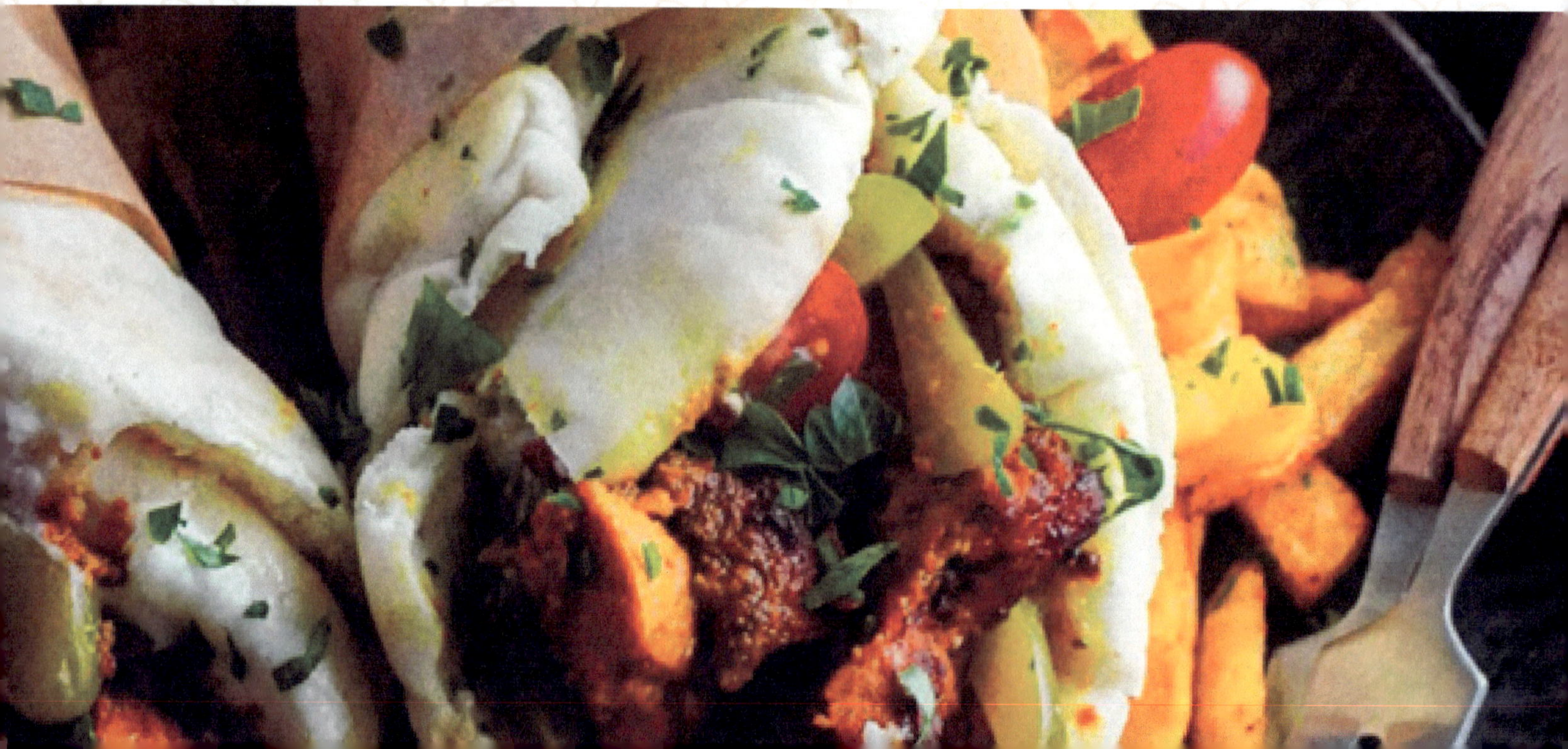

Koshari كشري

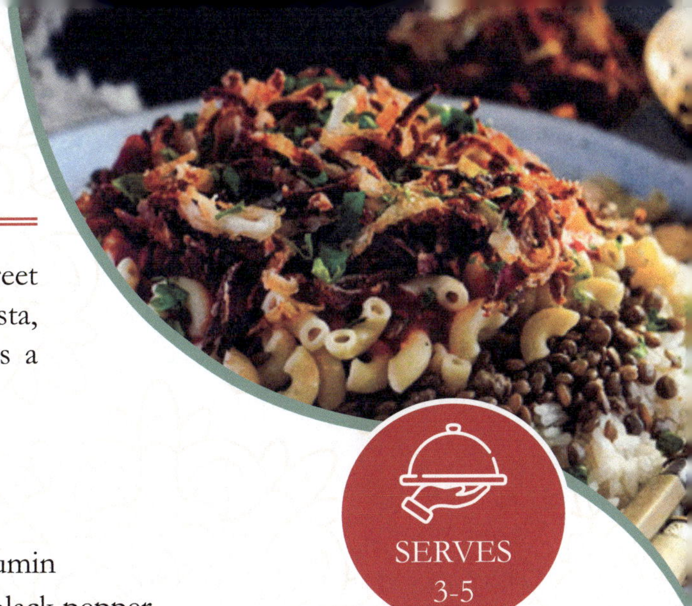

SERVES
3-5

Koshari Is the national dish of Egypt and a popular Egyptian street food. Essentially, it's Egyptian rice topped with spiced lentils, pasta, and a vinegary tomato sauce and crispy onions. The result is a delicious masterpiece.

INGREDIENTS:

Rice:

- 2 cups short grain rice, rinsed & soaked
- 3 tbsp oil
- 1 tsp salt
- 1 tsp ground cumin
- 3 cups boiling water
- 3 large yellow onions, fried
- 8 oz elbow pasta, cooked according to package instructions
- 15 oz can of hummus, rinsed & warmed

Lentils:

- 1 cup brown lentils, washed
- 1 tsp salt
- 1 tsp cumin
- ¼ tsp black pepper
- 3 cups hot water

Tomato Sauce:

- 1 tbsp oil
- 6 garlic cloves, minced
- 2 tbsp tomato paste
- 30 oz tomato sauce
- ½ tsp black pepper
- 1 tsp salt
- 1 tsp ground cumin
- 1 tbsp white vinegar

DIRECTIONS:

1. Wash and soak the rice for 20 minutes in cold water. Then, drain the excess water.
2. To start, slice the onions into thin wings and fry them in a generous amount of oil until they're golden brown. Transfer the onions to a paper towel to drain.
3. Drain and rinse the hummus, then warm it up. Cook the elbow pasta according to package instructions and set aside.

4. Add the washed lentils to a pot. Add the cumin, black pepper, and salt and mix. Top with the hot water and boil for 5 minutes, before simmering on medium-low heat until softened, about 20 minutes. Once cooked, drain any excess liquid.
5. To cook the rice, heat up 3 tablespoons of oil in a pot on high heat. In this case, I prefer using the oil used to fry the onions to add extra flavor. Add the drained rice, and saute until the rice grains are well coated in oil. Add the salt and cumin and mix well. Top it off with the boiling water and let the mixture boil for 5 minutes before reducing the heat to medium-low, and letting the rice simmer for 15-20 minutes, or until softened and cooked through.
6. To make the tomato sauce, heat up a tablespoon of oil on medium-high heat. Add the minced garlic and saute until golden. Now, add the tomato paste, and tomato sauce. Mix everything together well, then add the black pepper, salt, cumin, and vinegar. Let the mixture simmer on medium-low heat for 5 minutes or until hot and thickened.
7. To assemble, start with a layer of cooked rice, and top it off with cooked lentils. Now, add a layer of warmed hummus and cooked pasta. Top with the fried onions and tomato sauce.

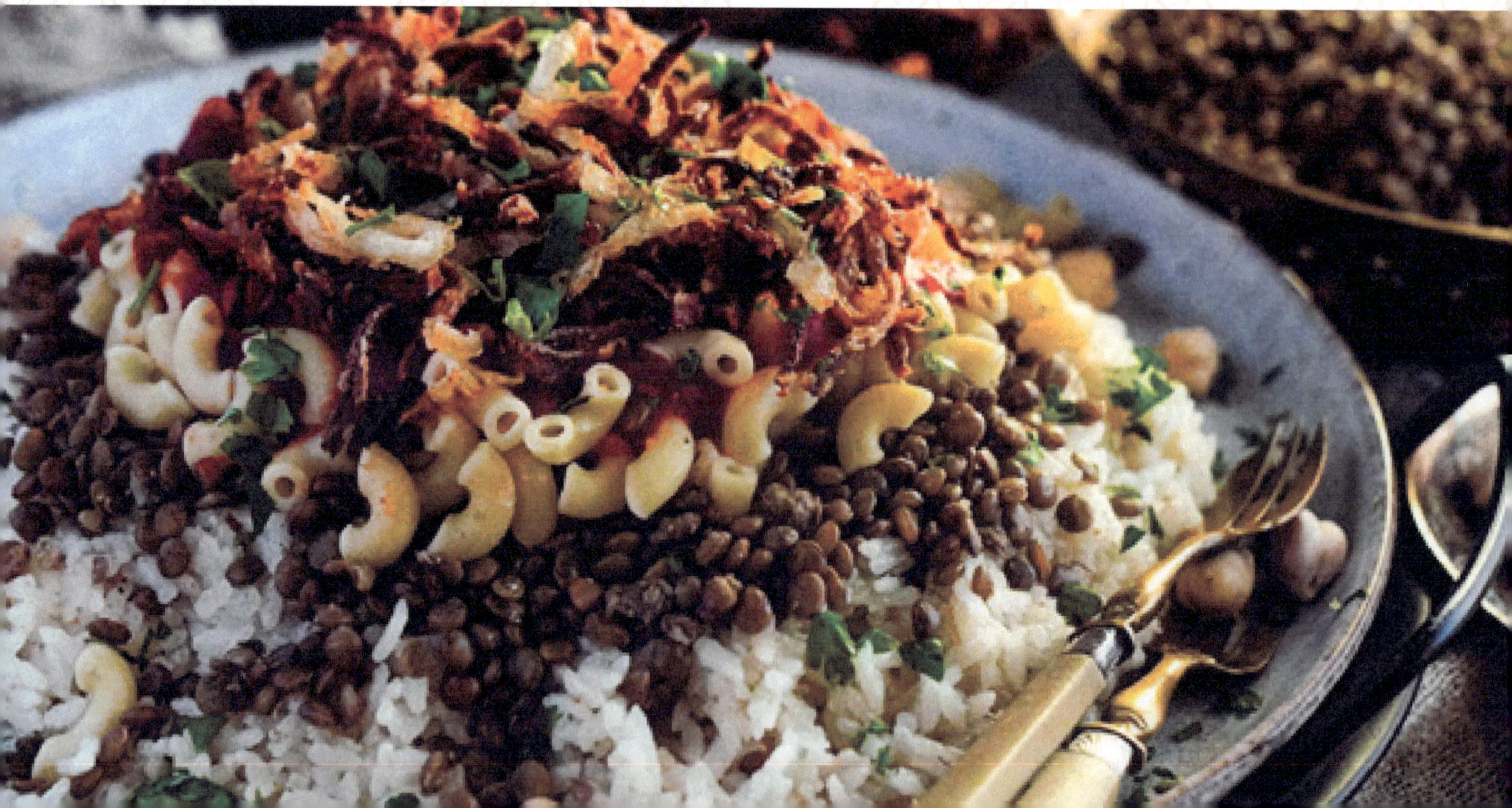

Haraa Osbao حراق اصبعه

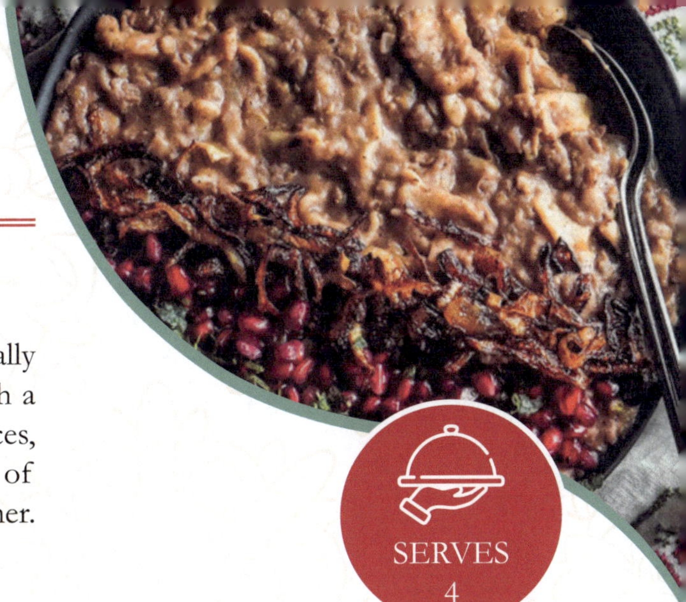

SERVES 4

(Syrian Pasta with Lentils & Caramelized Onions)

"Haraa Osbao" or "Harak Osbao" is a Syrian dish that typically consists of lentils and pasta cooked together and seasoned with a variety of spices. It is always topped with crunchy pita bread pieces, caramelized onions, and pomegranate seeds. It's packed full of protein and healthy nutrients, and it's the perfect side dish or dinner. It is very close to the Palestinian dish Rashta, or Irkak o Adas.

INGREDIENTS:

- 1 cup brown lentils
- 6 cups hot water
- 3 tbsp extra virgin olive oil
- 1 medium yellow onion, finely chopped
- 8 oz pasta, shape of choice
- 2 ½ tbsp pomegranate molasses
- 1 tsp cumin
- 1 ½ tsp 7 spices
- ½ tsp black pepper
- 1 tbsp bouillon powder
- 1 tsp sumac
- ½ tsp salt, or to taste

Garnish:

- Caramelized onions
- Pomegranate seeds
- Crunchy pita bread chunks
- Parsley or Cilantro

Pro Tip: Traditionally, fresh dough is made instead of using pasta. If you're up for it, combine 2 cups of all purpose flour and ¾ -1 cup water with a 1 teaspoon of salt until a cohesive and soft dough forms. Roll the dough thin onto a floured surface, and flour the top again. Cut into thin long strips, and add a light sprinkle of flour on top. Add this to the pot after sauteeing the onions, and let it cook for 5 minutes so the dough isn't raw.

DIRECTIONS:

1. Wash 1 cup of brown lentils and then boil them in 6 cups of water. Add 1 teaspoon of cumin, and ½ teaspoon of black pepper. Cook for 15-20 minutes or until the lentils are softened. Do not discard the liquid. Strain the lentils.

2. Meanwhile, cook your pasta according to package instructions. Drain.
3. In another pot, heat up the olive oil on medium-high heat.
4. Add the finely chopped onion and saute until golden, about 5 minutes.
5. Add in the strained and cooked lentils.
6. Add the 1 tablespoon of bouillon powder, 1 teaspoon sumac, and 1 ½ teaspoon 7 spices.
7. Add in the cooked and drained pasta, and the strained lentil liquid.
8. Adjust for salt, and let the mixture cook together for 5 minutes. If you'd like it less thick, add some hot water.
9. Serve, garnish with caramelized onions, crunchy pita bread chunks, pomegranate seeds and chopped parsley or cilantro to your liking.

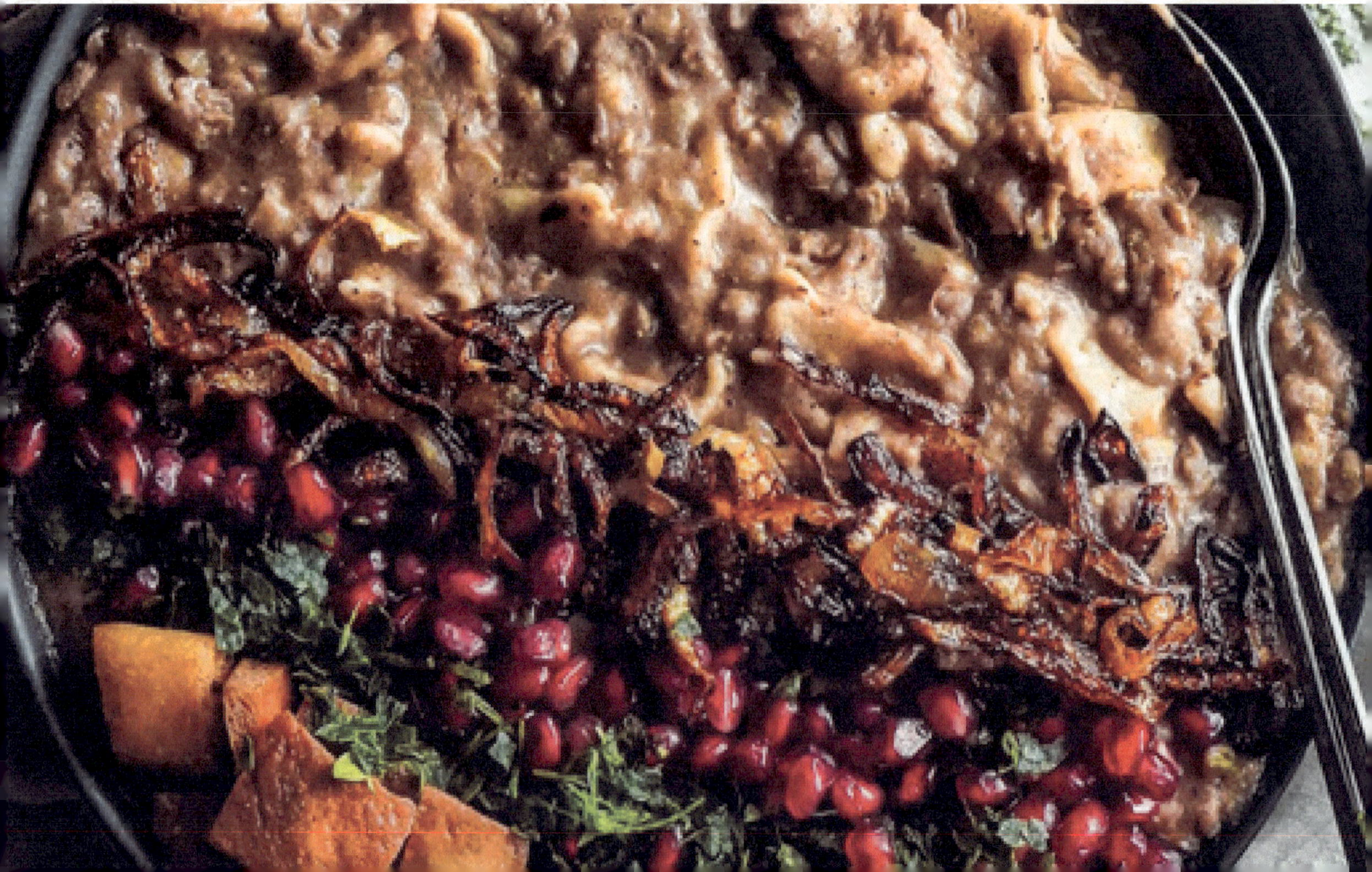

Lamb Makloubeh مقلوبة باللحمة

Makloubeh is a popular dish across the Levant that originated in Palestine, and its name literally means "upside down," because when the vegetables, rice, and lamb are layered into the pot and cooked, you flip the pot into a tray and the final dish looks like a layered cake. This makloubeh uses lamb and veggies, and it's absolutely delicious.

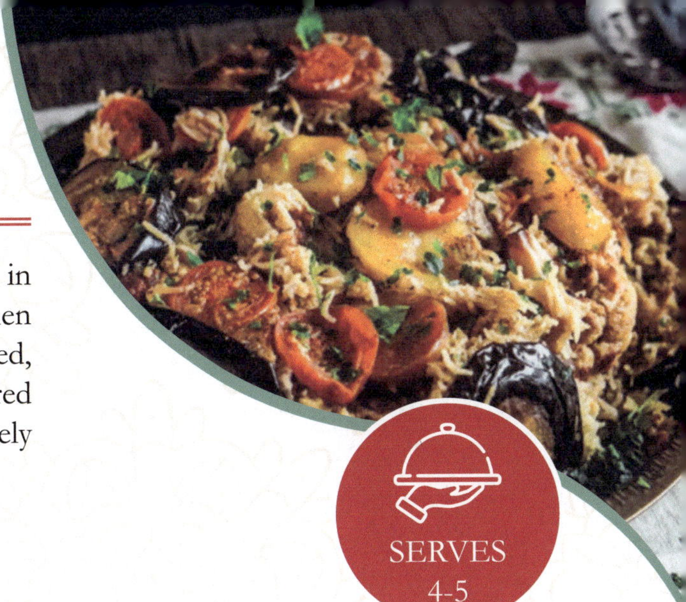

SERVES
4-5

INGREDIENTS:

For the Lamb Broth:

- 5 pieces bone-in lamb shoulder, about 4-5 lbs
- 5 garlic cloves
- ½ yellow onion
- 1 cinnamon stick
- 2 dried bay leaves
- 4 cardamom pods
- 1 tbsp7 spices
- 1 tsp coriander powder
- ½ tsp black pepper
- 2 tsp garlic powder
- 2 tsp onion powder
- ½ tsp turmeric,
- Salt, to taste

The Rice:

- 2 cups jasmine rice
- 2 tsp 7 spices
- 1 tsp coriander powder
- 1 tsp salt or to taste
- 4½ cups broth

Vegetables:

- 1 small cauliflower head
- 1 large eggplant
- 2 russet potatoes
- 1 cup baby carrots
- Tomatoes, for layering

DIRECTIONS:

Vegetable Prep:

1. Cut the cauliflower into single florets. You do not want really small pieces, think florets that are big enough to be picked up by a fork. Once cut, you want to deep fry until golden in color, about 10 minutes in hot oil.
2. Peel the eggplant and cut into 1 inch rounds. Place the rounds onto a clean kitchen towel or paper towels. Lightly salt both sides of the eggplant to dry out the moisture. Let it sit for 15 minutes before patting dry both sides. Once dried, fry until golden.
3. If you're using whole carrots, peel and cut them into quarter-inch thick pieces and about 2 inches in length. Deep fry until golden.

**I prefer using baby carrots to make it a little easier.*

4. Peel and cut the potato into ½ inch rounds. Deep fry until golden.
5. Once all the vegetables are fried, transfer to a strainer to drain excess oil.

The Lamb Broth:

1. Add the oil to a pot along with the whole garlic cloves and onion.
2. Saute until fragrant, and add the lamb. Saute until a little color develops, about 3-5 minutes and add the whole spices, and black pepper.
3. Add enough water to fully cover the lamb and let it boil for 15 minutes. Discard the liquid and whole spices. This gets rid of any scum or gaminess the lamb has.
4. Add the lamb back to the pot and add in the remaining powdered spices along with enough water to fully cover and submerge the lamb. Let it come to a rolling boil for 5 minutes before covering, and let it simmer for 45-60 minutes or until the lamb is fully cooked.
5. Once the lamb is fully cooked, set aside. Taste the broth and adjust for salt.
6. Strain the broth and set aside. Do not discard.

The Rice:

1. Wash the rice thoroughly. Submerge with cold water and let it soak for 30 minutes. Drain.
2. Add the spices to the drained rice and mix.

Layering:

1. Begin by adding a piece of parchment paper around the same size as the bottom of your pot. Add sliced tomatoes.
2. Add the cooked lamb on top, making sure to lay the pieces side by side.
3. Add the fried vegetables. Make sure to lay them flat all around the pot to ensure everything is even.
4. Add the seasoned rice on top of the vegetables.
5. Finally, add the strained broth on top. It is preferred to heat up the broth before adding it on top of the rice.
6. Let the pot come to a boil on high heat. Let it boil for 5 minutes.
7. Cover with aluminum foil and the pot cover and lower the heat to medium-low. Let it simmer for 30-40 minutes, or until the rice is cooked.
8. To make sure it keeps shape when flipped, let the pot rest for 15-20 minutes after it is finished cooking. Then, flip onto a serving platter.
9. Top with toasted almonds if desired, and serve with yogurt and Arabic salad.

Pro Tips:

- You can omit a vegetable you dislike. Some variations also use cooked chickpeas as well.
- You can fry or air fry your vegetables the day before to give yourself a head start!
- Add parchment paper the same size as the bottom of your pot before you begin layering to help prevent sticking and scorching!
- To ensure it keeps the beautiful layered shape once flipped, use a pot with flat handles. This way it lays flat onto the serving platter you'll flip onto.

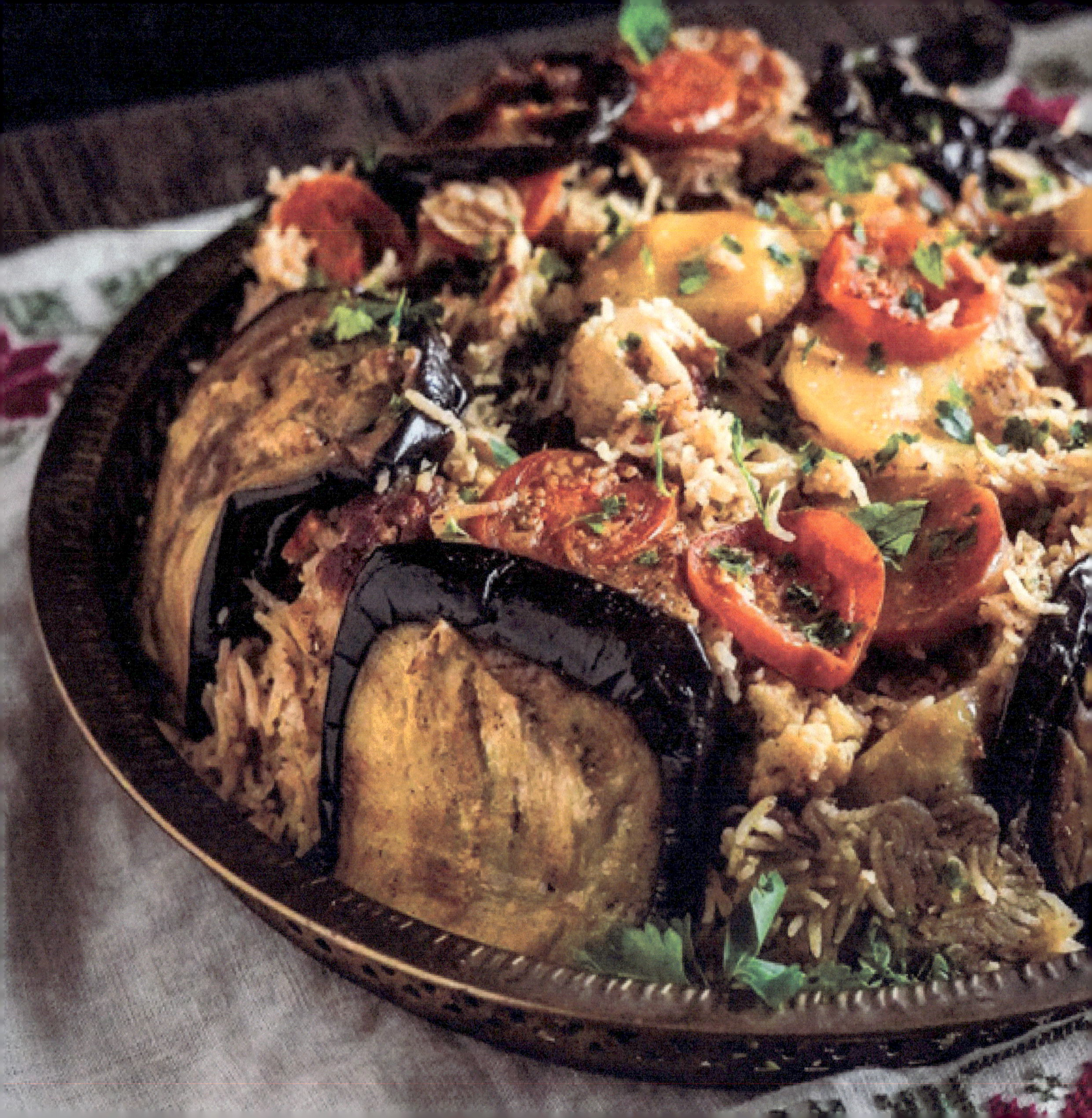

Middle Eastern Whole Baked Fish سمك مشوي

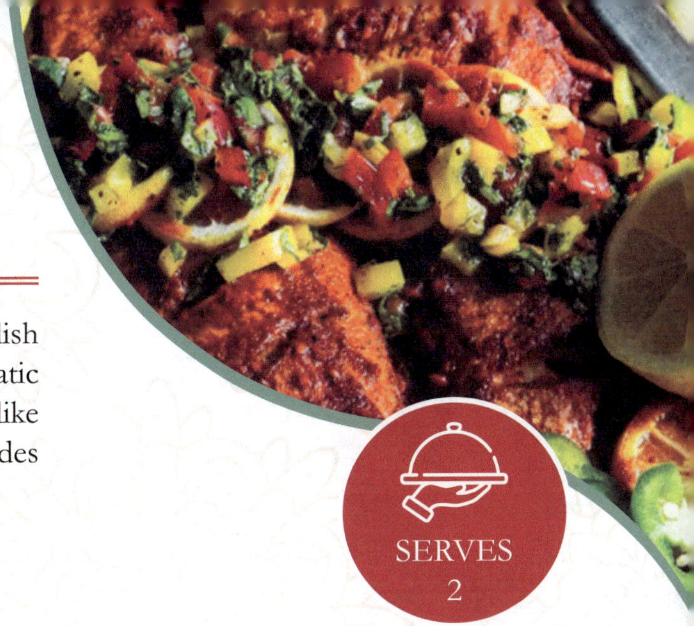

Middle Eastern whole baked fish is a delicious and flavorful dish that showcases the region's love for fresh seafood and aromatic spices. The preparation often involves seasoning a whole fish like red snapper, and baking it to perfection. It can be served with sides of rice, salad, and a variety of sauces.

SERVES
2

INGREDIENTS:

- 2 whole red snappers, cleaned and descaled
- 1 tsp sumac
- 2 tbsp red pepper paste
- 2 garlic cloves, minced
- 3 tbsp extra virgin olive oil
- ½ tsp cumin
- 1 tsp 7 spices
- 2 tsp salt, or to taste
- 1 tsp coriander powder
- ¼ tsp black pepper
- 2 lemon slices

DIRECTIONS:

1. Preheat the oven to 425 F.
2. Score each fish to make 3 slits in each fish.
3. In a bowl, combine together the minced garlic, extra virgin olive oil, and the seasonings along with the red pepper paste.
4. Add the spice paste to the fish, making sure to season the inside of the fish as well.
5. Place the fish on a baking sheet lined with parchment paper.
6. Add a lemon slice on top of each fish.
7. Bake at 425 F for about 20 minutes, or until the eyes pop out and the flesh is firm to the touch.

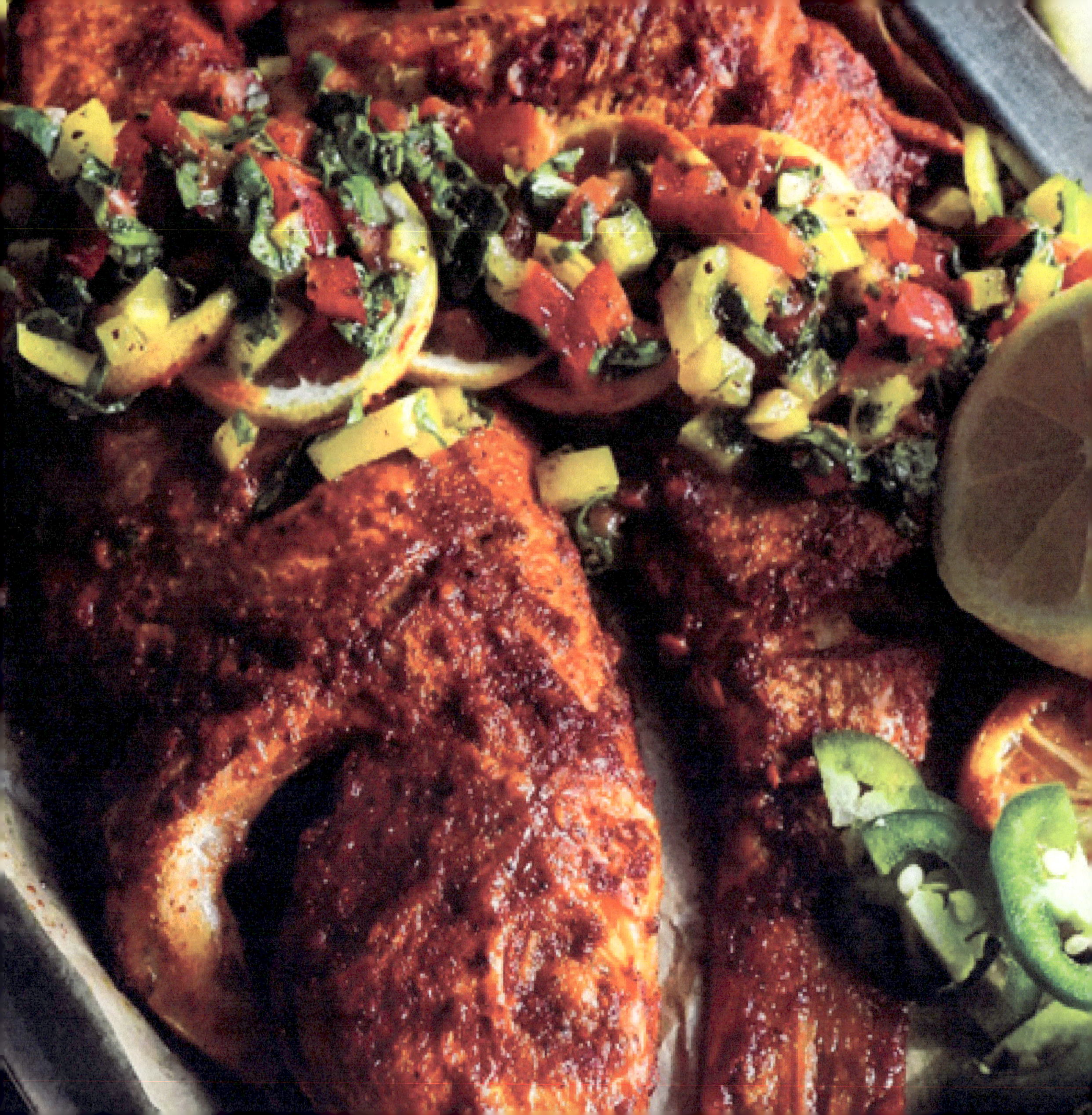

One Pot Ouzi Rice أرز الأوزي

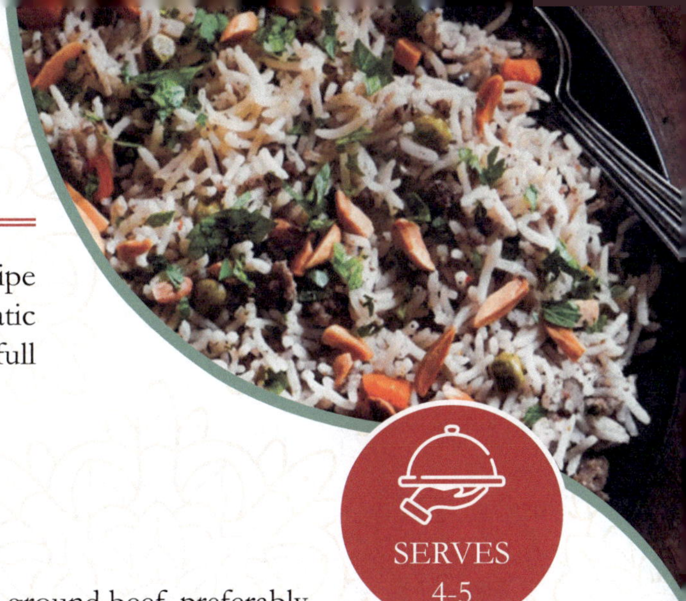

SERVES 4-5

Ouzi rice with ground beef is a traditional Middle Eastern recipe made with well-seasoned basmati rice, peas and carrots, aromatic beef, and toasted nuts. This well-balanced dish is delicious and full of nutrients, and this is a quicker way to make it with less mess.

INGREDIENTS:

The Rice:

- 1½ cups basmati rice, soaked and washed
- 1 cup frozen carrots and peas
- 2 tsp 7 spices
- 1½ tsp coriander powder
- 1 tsp Aleppo pepper (optional)
- 1½ tsp salt (or to taste)
- ½ tsp turmeric
- ¼ tsp cinnamon
- 3 cups hot water

The Beef:

- ¾ pound ground beef, preferably 80% lean
- 2 tbsp extra virgin olive oil
- 1 medium yellow onion, diced
- 3 garlic cloves, minced
- ¾ tsp 7 spices
- ¾ tsp coriander powder
- 1 tsp salt
- ½ tsp black pepper
- ½ tsp cinnamon

DIRECTIONS:

1. Begin by soaking and washing the basmati rice. Soak for 20 minutes in cold water, then drain.
2. To start making the beef, add the olive oil to a pot on medium-high heat. Add the onion and saute until translucent, about 5 minutes or so. Add the minced garlic and saute until fragrant.
3. Add the ground beef and let it heat up for a few minutes. Begin breaking up the large chunks into small ones using your spatula. Cook until completely browned.
4. Add the ¾ teaspoon 7 spices, ¾ teaspoon coriander powder, teaspoon of salt,½ teaspoon of black pepper, and ½ teaspoon of cinnamon. Saute until the ground beef is well seasoned.
5. Add frozen or thawed carrots and peas and cook until warmed, about 3-4 minutes.
6. Add the previously washed and drained rice.

7. Add the remaining 7 spices, coriander powder, cinnamon, salt, and turmeric. Mix well.
8. Pour 3 cups of hot water on top and stir.
9. Once it starts boiling, let it boil for 2-3 minutes before covering, and lowering the heat to low.
10. Cook for 15-20 minutes or until the rice is fluffy.
11. Garnish with chopped parsley and toasted almond slivers. Serve with salad and yogurt.

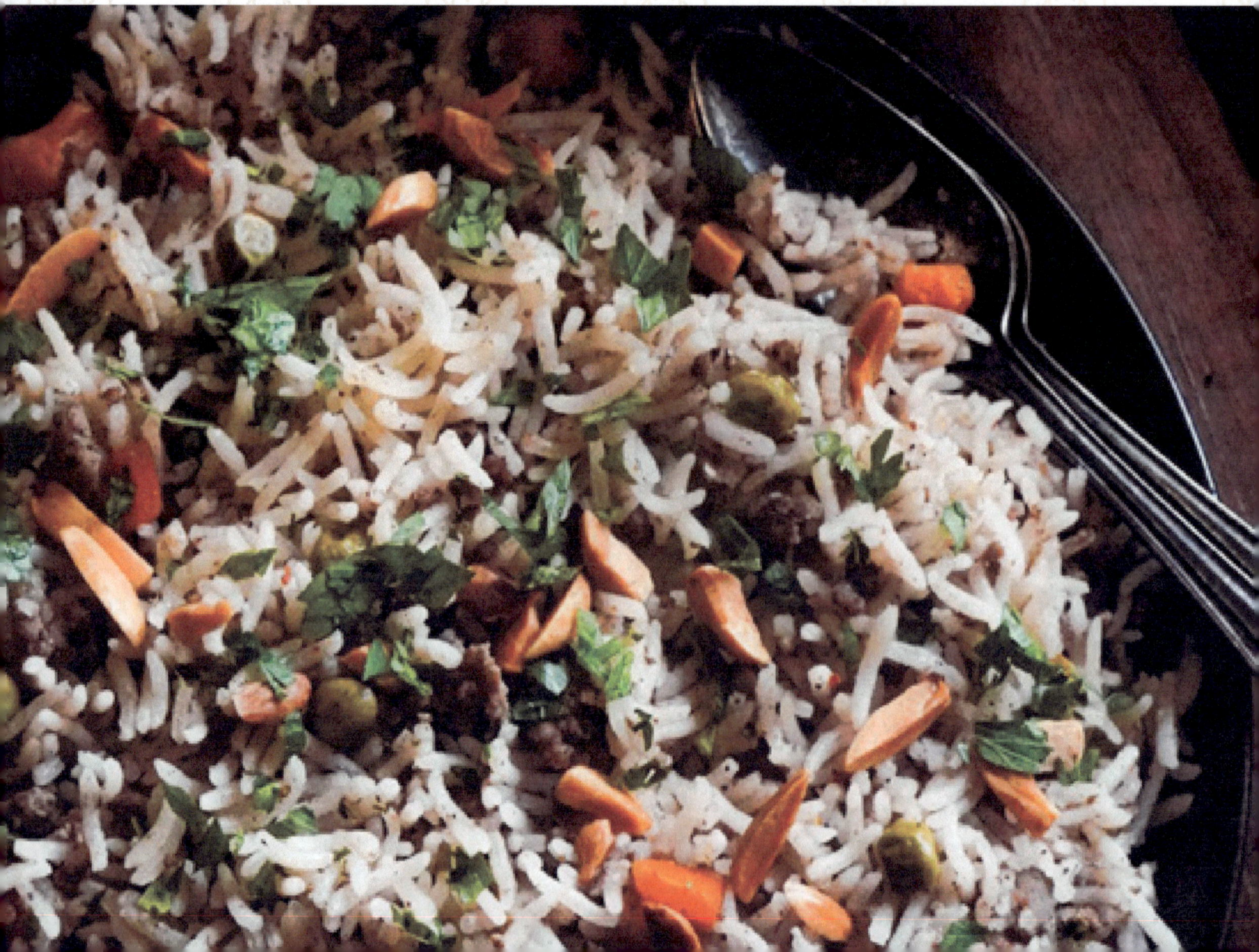

Middle Eastern Roasted Leg of Lamb فخذة خروف مشوية

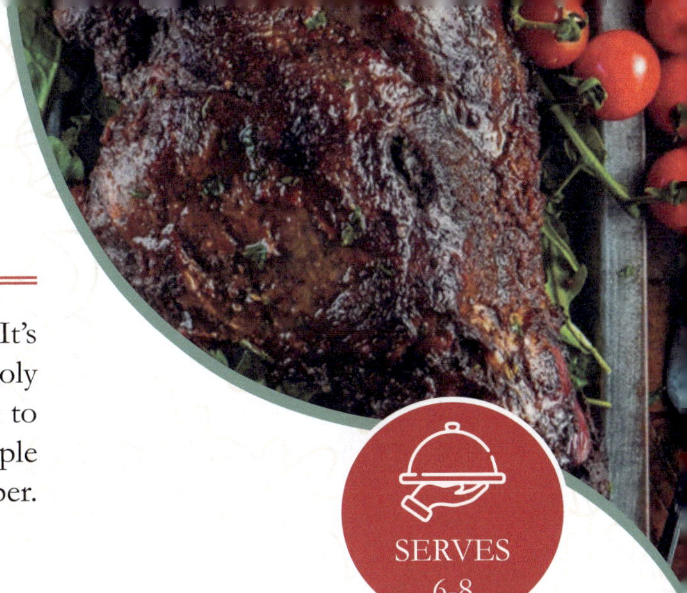

Lamb is a common Middle Eastern household staple protein. It's used in a variety of rice dishes, and in most stews. During the holy month of Ramadan, or any special occasion, people often opt to make a roasted leg of lamb for its ease in feeding multiple people at once. Also, for how it looks because it's definitely a showstopper.

SERVES 6-8

INGREDIENTS:

The Marinade:

- Leg of lamb, about 7-9 lbs
- 1 roma tomato
- ½ yellow onion
- 8 cloves garlic
- ½ cup yogurt
- 1 tbsp mustard
- 2 tsp salt
- ½ tsp black pepper
- ½ a red bell pepper
- 2 tsp 7 spices
- 2 tsp garlic powder
- 1½ tsp onion powder

To Serve:

- 1 tsp saffron threads
- 2 tbsp unsalted butter, melted

DIRECTIONS:

1. Trim off the big chunks of excess fat on the leg of lamb. Do not remove all fat, just the big and thick pockets of it.
2. Pat dry the lamb on all sides using a paper towel
3. Using a sharp knife, poke holes through the lamb about an inch deep making sure to poke them on every side of the lamb.
4. To a food processor, add the garlic, onion, bell pepper, and tomato, and make sure they're completely puréed.
5. Add the spices, yogurt, mustard, and olive oil to the mixture and mix well.

6. Pour the spice and vegetable mixture all over the leg of lamb and massage it through, making sure it gets into the crevices you created.
7. Cover and let it marinate for 12+ hours.
8. Bake covered in a preheated oven at 350 for 4-5 hours (you might need longer).
9. Bloom the saffron threads in a tablespoon of hot water for 10 minutes.
10. Mix the saffron with the melted butter, and brush all over the cooked lamb.

Serve with ouzi rice, salads, and yogurt.

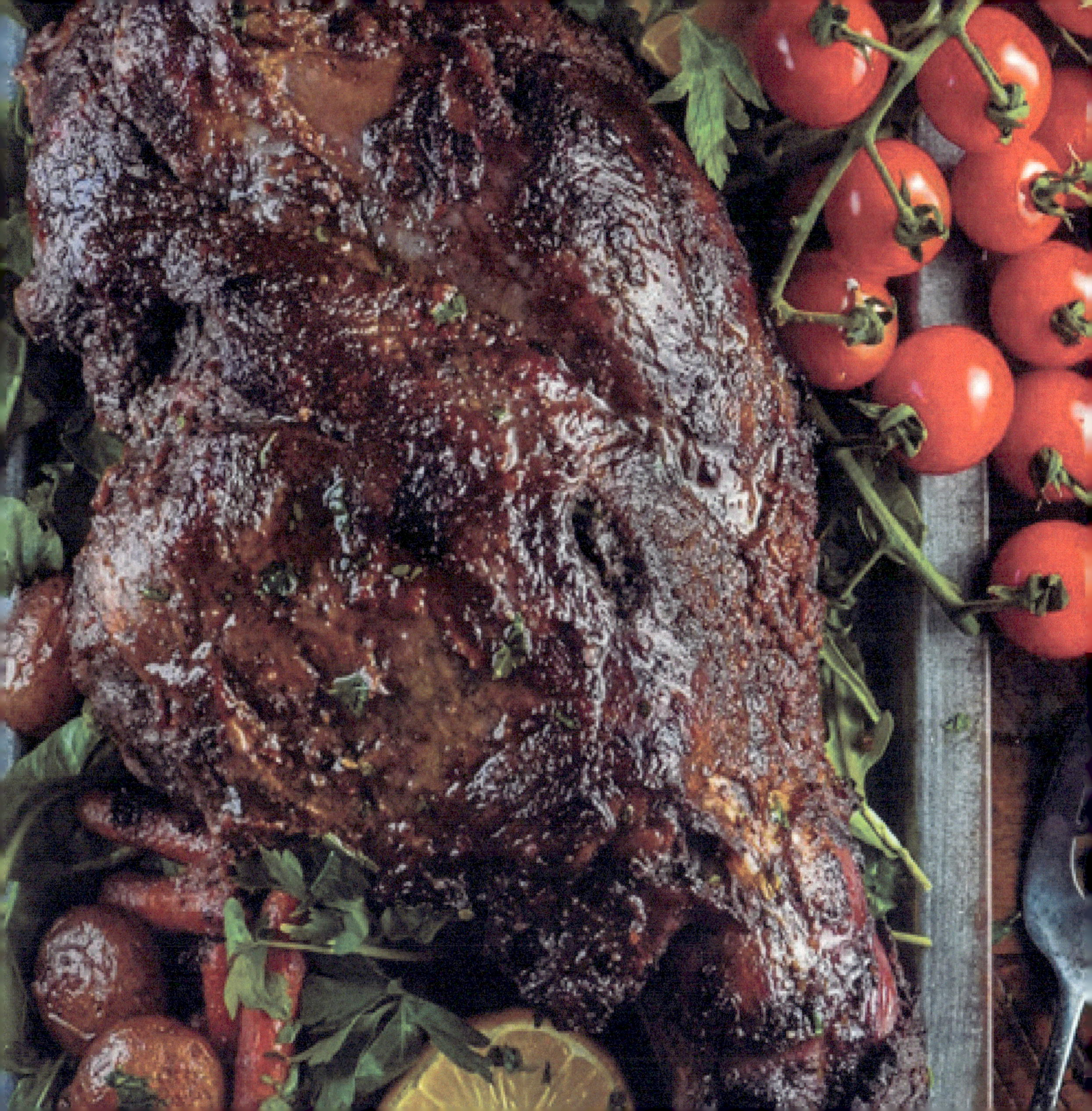

Musakhan مسخن

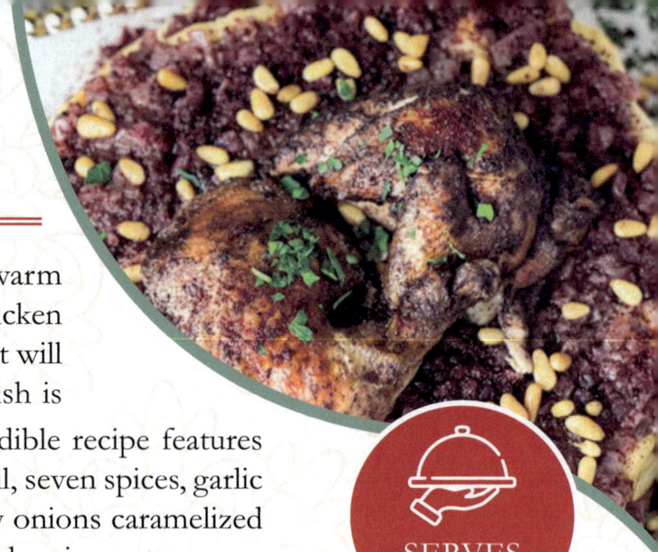

Traditional Palestinian Musakhan Recipe is the epitome of a warm cozy chicken dish. It is a warm-your-heart juicy Middle Eastern chicken meal that is flavor-packed with sumac and caramelized onions. It will definitely dazzle your taste buds. This traditional Palestinian dish is known far and wide as a national Palestinian plate. This incredible recipe features tender chicken marinated in an aromatic blend of sumac, olive oil, seven spices, garlic powder, ground coriander, and salt. It is then brought to life by onions caramelized to perfection with sumac and olive oil, finally topped with crunchy pine nuts.

SERVES 6-8

INGREDIENTS:

Musakhan

- 8 large red onions, medium chop
- 2 cups extra virgin olive oil
- Chicken bullion powder to taste
- ⅓ cup sumac
- Pine nuts, fried or toasted
- Taboon or plain naan bread

Musakhan Chicken

- 3 small chickens
- ¼ cup extra virgin olive oil
- 1 tbsp sumac
- 1 tbsp 7 spices
- 1 tbsp ground coriander
- 1 tbsp garlic powder
- 2 tbsp salt

DIRECTIONS:

1. Preheat the oven to 450 F.
2. Chicken for Musakhan is cut either into 2 halves (of a whole chicken) or into 4 pieces. Then, pat it dry with a paper towel.
3. Mix the sumac, 7 spices, coriander powder, garlic powder, and salt together with the olive oil, then brush onto each chicken piece from all sides. Place onto a baking sheet lined with parchment paper, making sure the chicken is not tightly packed so it has enough room to crisp up.
4. Cover with aluminum foil, and bake for about 1 hour, then uncover and bake for an additional 15-20 minutes, so the skin gets crispy and develops a golden-brown color

5. Cut the onions and sauté in a pot on low heat. Keep mixing until the onions become soft, have a bright pink color to them, and have released all their water.
6. Continue sauteing, and add the sumac and bouillon powder. Let it continue cooking on low for an additional 5 minutes, or until the onions are no longer crunchy.
7. Start with 1 Naan or Taboon. Using a slotted spoon, take some onions and spread on top. Depending on the size of your bread, add enough to reach the edges but not so much that it piles up in the middle.
8. Sprinkle some sumac all around the onions and add some fried pine nuts.
9. Serve each chicken on a bread piece topped for one person or layer multiple bread pieces on top of each other. Then, add the chicken on the final top layer.

Pro Tips:

» Using good quality sumac ensures a delicious tangy flavor. If you're not using good quality sumac, you might need to add a splash of lemon or citric acid.

» Add the boullion slowly, to not make it salty. Adding the bouillon powder here instead of salt gives a more balanced flavor profile.

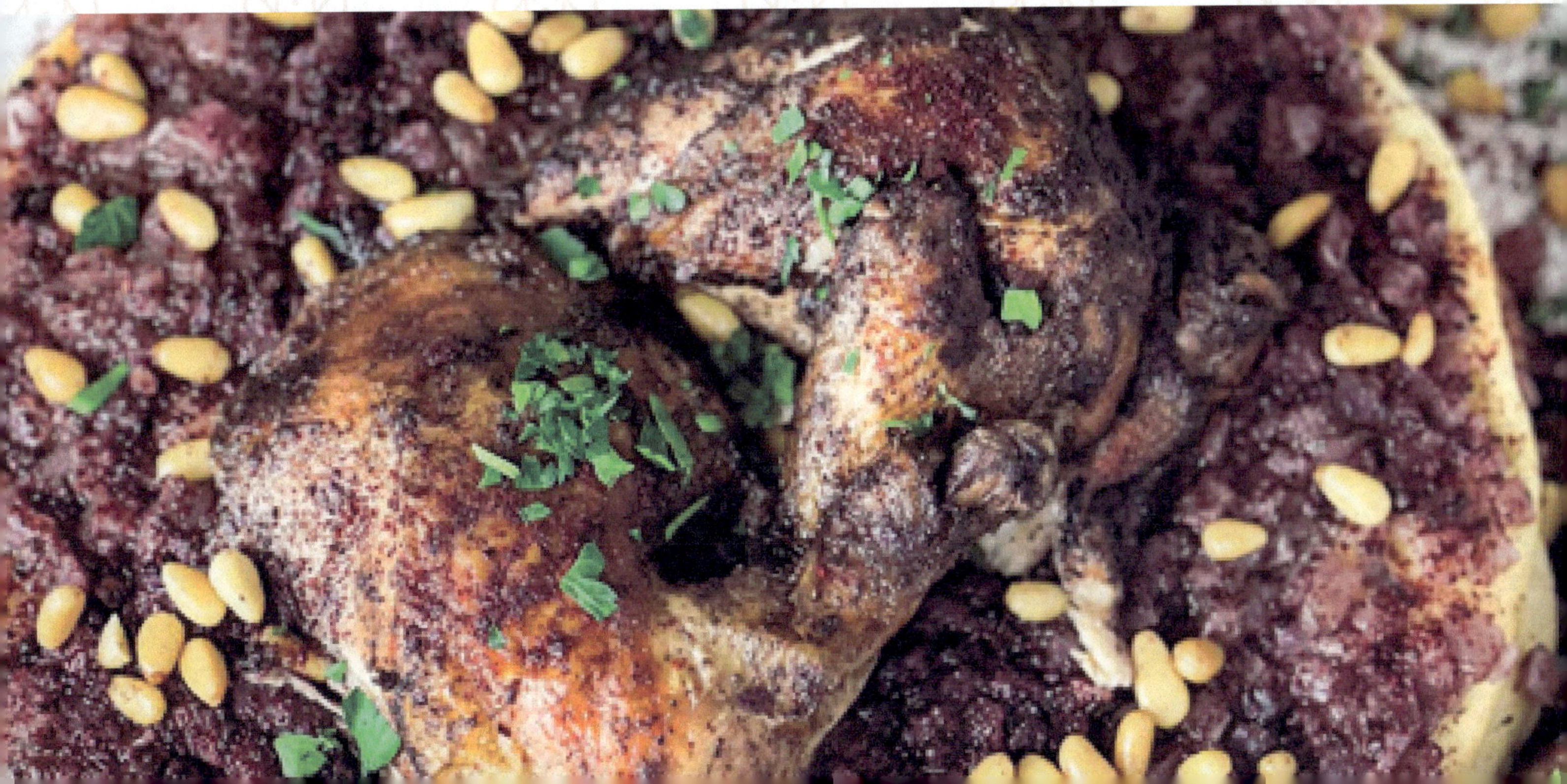

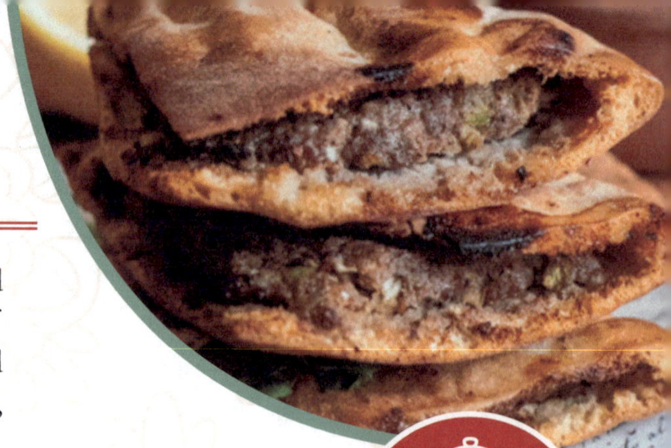

Arayes عرايس

Arayes is a popular Middle Eastern dish that consists of grilled or baked stuffed pita bread filled with a seasoned mixture of minced meat. It's a flavorful and satisfying dish that is enjoyed in various Middle Eastern countries like Palestine, Jordan, Syria, and Lebanon. In Egypt, it is referred to as hawawshi.

SERVES

INGREDIENTS:

- 1 small yellow onion
- 1 lb ground beef, 80%
- 1 lb ground beef, 90% lean
- 4 garlic cloves
- 2 large roma tomatoes (250g)
- ¾ a bell pepper
- ⅓ jalapeno (optional)
- 2 tsp Aleppo pepper
- 2 tsp 7 spices
- 1 tbsp salt
- ½ tsp black pepper
- 3 tbsp of extra virgin olive oil, plus more for brushing.

DIRECTIONS:

1. Add the vegetables to a food processor and process until chunky.
2. Add to the beef along with the spices and mix well.
3. Fill into your pita, to your desired thickness. Do not make them too thick or they won't cook fully and evenly.
4. Brush a small amount of olive oil (about 1 teaspoon) on each side of the pita.
5. Grill or bake at 425°F until the beef is all the way cooked through and the bread is crispy (about 8-10 minutes per side depending on your oven). Or you can air fry on 400°F for 12-16 minutes flipping halfway.

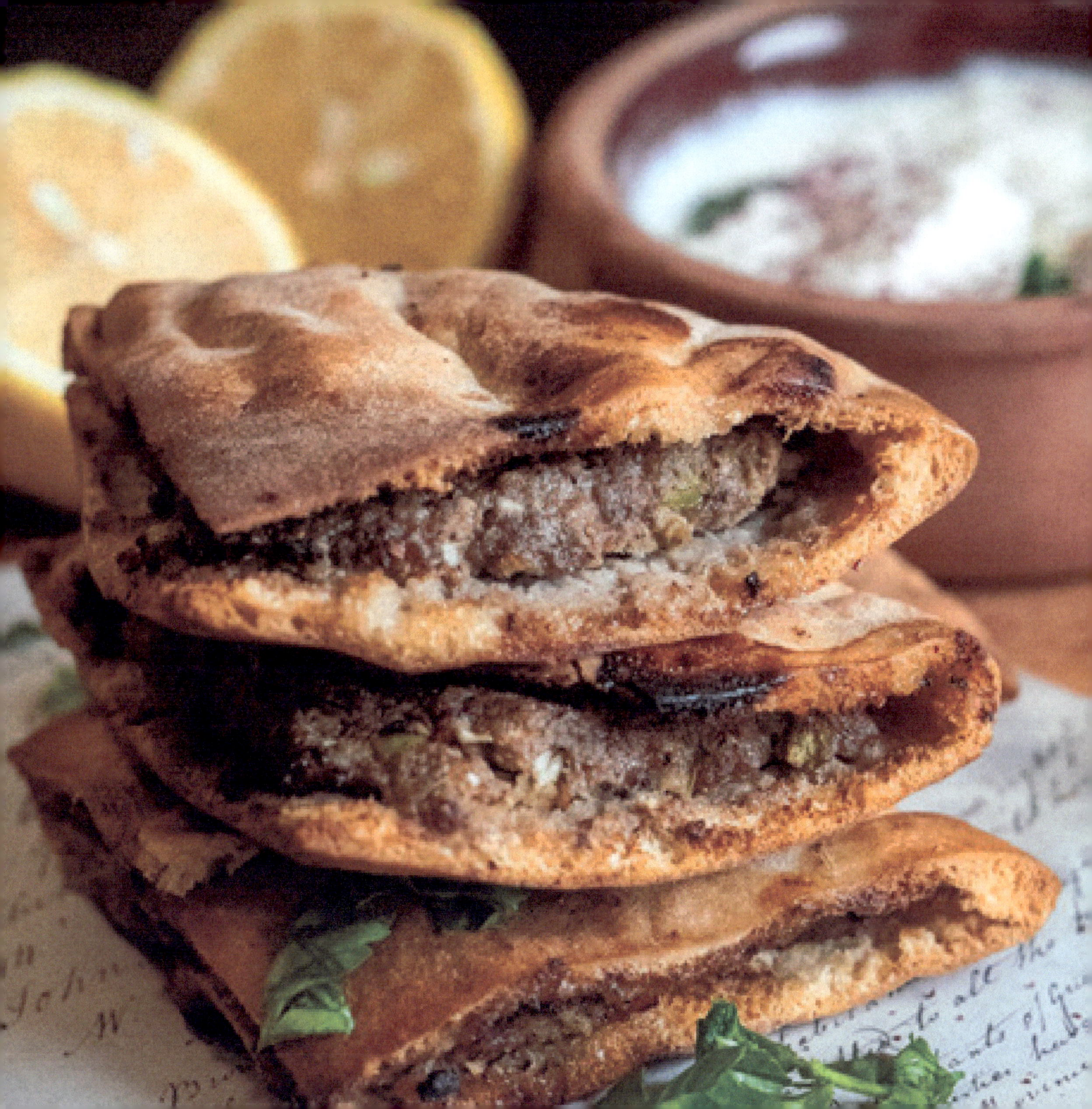

Burghul Stuffed Peppers

فليفلة محشية بالبرغل

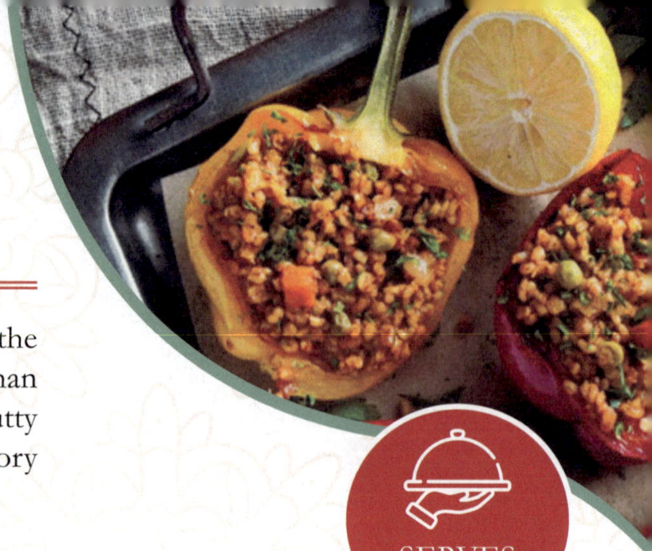

SERVES
3-4

Stuffed Peppers are a common dish across many cuisines. In the Arab world, it would most often be stuffed with a grain rather than a protein. In this case, the bulgur adds a beautiful light and nutty taste, and combined with the seasonings, it offers a delicious, savory meal.

INGREDIENTS:

For the Filling:

- 4 red or orange bell peppers
- 1 ¼ cup coarse burghul (bulgur), washed
- 3 tbsp extra virgin olive oil, divided
- 1 medium yellow onion, finely chopped
- 8 garlic cloves, minced
- 1 roma tomato, finely chopped
- ½ cup frozen peas and carrots mix
- 2 cups hot water

Seasonings:

- 1 tbsp tomato paste
- 1 tbsp mild pepper paste
- ¼ tsp Aleppo pepper
- ¼ tsp turmeric
- ¼ tsp cumin
- ¼ tsp black pepper
- 2 tsp bouillon powder
- 1 ½ tsp 7 spices
- ½ tsp salt
- 2 tbsp lemon juice

DIRECTIONS:

1. Preheat the oven to 425 F.
2. Cut the peppers in half, remove the inner seeds. Coat the peppers with 1 tbsp of the olive oil. Sprinkle them with salt and pepper. Add to a baking sheet lined with parchment paper and bake for 20 minutes, flipping halfway.
3. Wash the bulgur thoroughly, about 3-4 times. Drain the excess water.

4. Heat the 2 tablespoons of olive oil in a pot on high heat. Add the diced onion and garlic. Saute until golden, then add the chopped tomatoes and the peas and carrots. Saute for 2-3 minutes, until softened. Add in the tomato and pepper paste and mix. Now, add in the washed bulgur along with the seasonings and mix well.
5. Add the 2 cups of hot water and mix well, letting it come to a boil for 2-3 minutes. Once boiling, reduce the heat to medium-low and cover. Let it simmer for 15 minutes before fluffing with a fork.
6. Once the peppers are done cooking, stuff each half with the cooked bulgur and serve with yogurt or chopped Arabic salad.

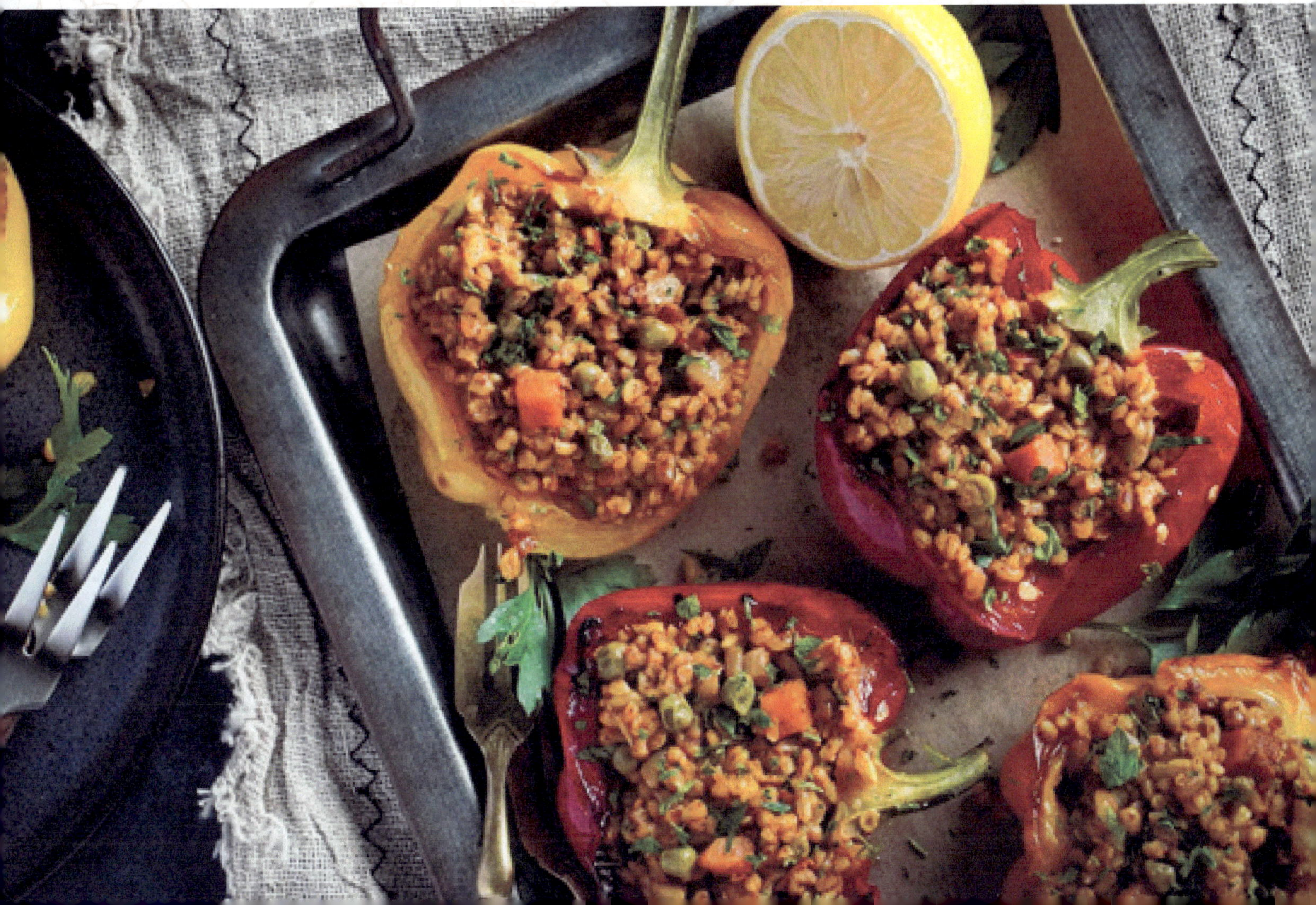

Chicken Zurbian زربيان الدجاج

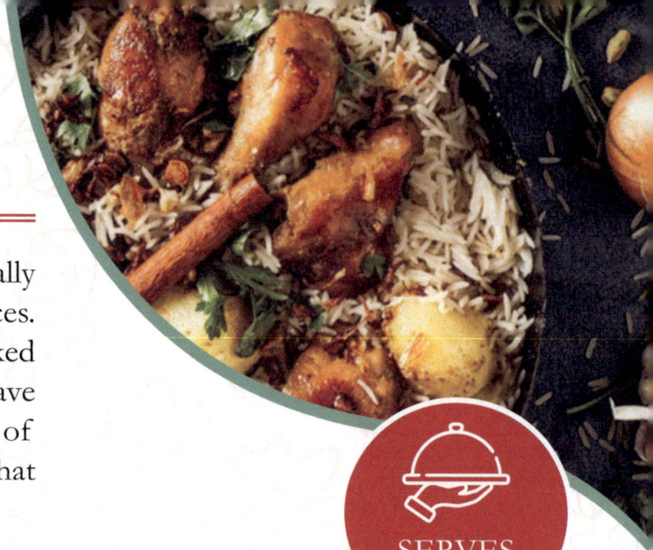

This authentic Yemeni dish is prepared by cooking protein, usually lamb or chicken, with a sauce of tomato, yogurt, and spices. The rice is placed on top of the meat, and it is typically cooked underground, in an oven called a Tannour. My husband and I have an obsession with trying new Yemeni dishes, and this one is one of our favorites. The chicken and rice are so flavorful and fragrant that you'll absolutely love it.

SERVES 4

INGREDIENTS:

- 2.5 lbs bone in, skinless chicken thighs and drumsticks
- 1.5 large yellow onions, cut into thin wings
- 5 whole baby potatoes, peeled (if they're large, cut in half)
- 5 garlic cloves
- 3/4 cup yogurt
- 2 tbsp ginger paste or 1 inch fresh ginger, finely chopped
- 1 tsp ground cumin, ground coriander, turmeric, and ground cardamom
- 1/2 tsp ground cinnamon
- 1/2 tsp black pepper
- 2 dried bay leaves
- 1 cinnamon stick
- 4 cardamom pods
- 2 tbsp oil

The Rice:

- 1 cup basmati rice, soaked for 20 minutes and rinsed
- 2 cups water, to parboil
- 1 cinnamon stick
- 5 whole cloves
- 4 cardamom pods

DIRECTIONS:

1. Cut the onions into thin wings and fry in hot oil until caramelized. The onions need to be brown and crispy. Once fried, set aside on a paper towel to absorb excess oil.
2. In a blender or food processor, add 1/2 of the fried onions along with the yogurt, garlic cloves, fresh ginger or ginger paste, and the ground spices. Blend until smooth. Pour the mixture over the skinless chicken and the cut potatoes. Marinate for a minimum of 30 minutes.

3. To a pot, add 2 tablespoons of the oil you used to fry the onions in. Once heated, add the marinated chicken and potatoes. Now, add the 2 bay leaves, 4 cardamom pods, and the cinnamon stick. Cook on medium-high until the chicken is completely golden, and no longer pink. Cover while cooking. This can take 20-30 minutes. Stir constantly so they don't stick or burn.
4. In the meantime, in another pot, add 3 cups of water along with 1 cinnamon stick, 5 whole cloves, and 4 cardamom pods. Let it come to a rolling boil. Add the washed and drained basmati rice. Stir. Let the rice cook on high for 5-10 minutes, it should be about 3/4 cooked through. Drain the rice and set aside. Once the chicken and the rice are fully cooked, you're ready to assemble.
5. Check to make sure there isn't too much liquid from the chicken. You don't want it to be watery, as this makes the rice mushy. If there's too much liquid, drain the excess.
6. Once the chicken is ready, you're going to add half of your drained rice on top. Add 1/2 of your remaining onions, then top with the remaining amount of rice. Cover and lower the heat to low. Let it steam for 15 minutes.
7. Once 15 minutes are up, light a piece of charcoal and place it inside a heat proof bowl or foil pocket on top of the rice. Add a drop of oil, and watch the charcoal smoke. Immediately cover the pot with the lid and let the dish absorb the smokiness for 10 minutes.
8. Remove the charcoal and fluff the rice. Transfer to a serving dish and top with caramelized onions and parsley.
9. Serve with Sahawiq and Yogurt.

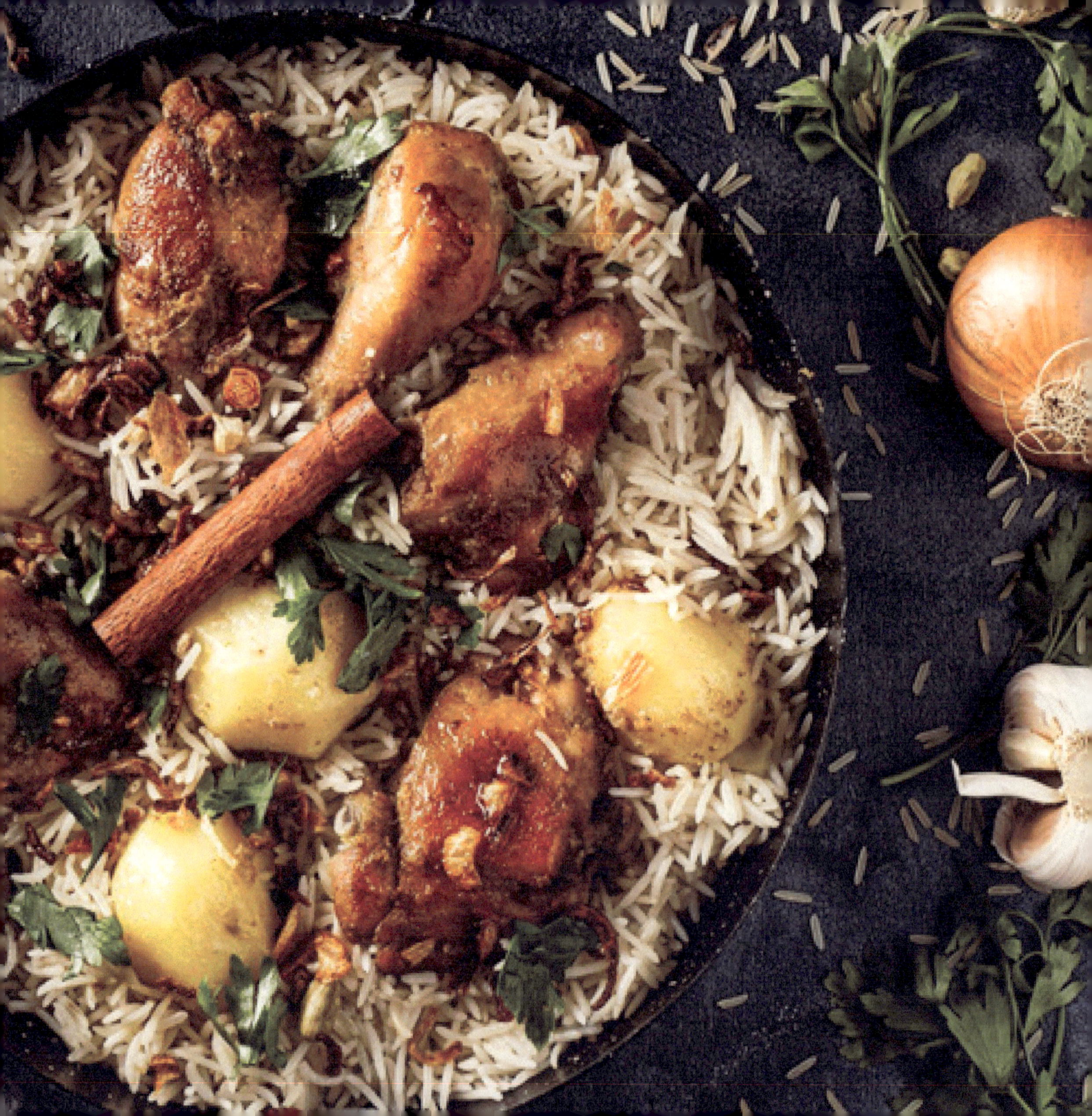

Dawali (Stuffed Grape Leaves) دوالي باللحمة

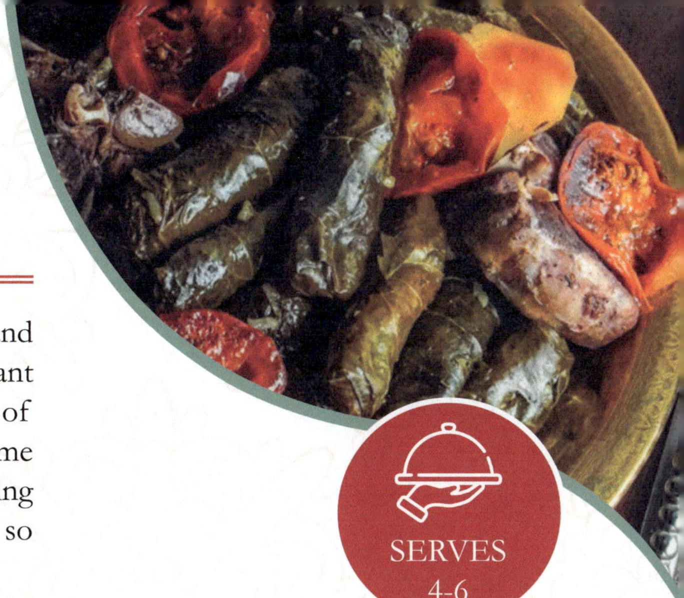

SERVES 4-6

Stuffed grape leaves, often referred to as Dawali by Palestinians and Jordanians, are delicious cooked leaves with an aromatic, fragrant filling of beef or lamb. They're usually accompanied by pieces of tender lamb in the pot. There are many variations of Dawali. Some make it vegetarian, and some make it with the filling only using protein and rice. This recipe is my mother's and everyone loves it so I'm positive you will too.

INGREDIENTS:

For the Filling:

- 1 jar Al-Afia grape leaves, rinsed and drained (16oz, 454g)
- 2.5 cups calrose or sushi rice, washed and soaked
- ½ lb 80/20% lean ground beef
- ½ medium yellow onion
- 2 large tomatoes
- ¼ cup fresh mint
- 8 cloves garlic
- 1 bunch parsley
- 1 tbsp 7 spices
- 1 ½ tsp coriander powder
- 1 ½ tsp bouillon powder
- 1/2 tsp ground cardamom
- 1/4 tsp black pepper
- 1 tsp turmeric
- 1 tsp salt or more to taste
- ¼ cup extra virgin olive oil
- 3 tbsp lemon juice

For the Lamb:

- 8 lamb chops or lamb loin chops (about 1 ½ - 2 lbs)
- 2 tbsp extra virgin olive oil
- 1 tsp 7 spice

To Assemble:

- 2 large tomatoes, cut into ¼-½ inch circles
- 8 pieces of lamb chops, or loin chops
- 2 tbsp olive oil
- 2 tbsp bouillon powder
- 4 ½ cups boiling water
- 2 tbsp lemon juice

DIRECTIONS:

1. To start, thoroughly wash the rice then let it soak for 20 minutes, and discard the excess liquid.
2. Finely chop the parsley, onion, garlic, tomatoes, and mint. Alternatively, you can pulse them in a food processor until chunky, but not liquidy.
3. Mix the chopped vegetables with the soaked and drained rice. Now add ground beef or lamb, lemon juice, and the seasonings. Mix together well.
4. To stuff the leaves, flatten one grape leaf on a cutting board or clean surface. Add about 1-2 tablespoons of the filling to the side of the leaf that's textured, not smooth. Add the filling at the bottom of the leaf, near the stem. If the stem is attached, cut it off. Spread the filling like a thin log along the edge of the bottom of the leaf. Now, fold the left and right side of the leaf towards the middle, to cover the filling. Now roll from the bottom to the top tightly, like rolling a burrito or cigar.
5. Before layering the Dawali pot, I prefer searing the lamb until it develops a crust and is no longer gamey. To do so, heat up 2 tbsp of olive oil in a pan. Sprinkle the lamb with the 7 spices and sear on both sides until browned and a nice crust develops, this can take 3-5 minutes per side.
6. To a heavy bottom pot, add the sliced tomatoes to line the bottom. Add the seared lamb. Now, layer the stuffed and rolled grape leaves one by one, making sure to get them all around the pot. Stack until the'yre finished. Make sure you use a large pot that fits.
7. Next, transfer the pot to the stove on high heat. Add the bouillon powder to the boiling water, along with the lemon juice and olive oil. You want the water to be 1 ½ inches above the rolled leaves, so if you need more water, go ahead and add it. Let it come to a rolling boil for 5 minutes, before lowering the heat to medium-low. Cover with aluminum foil, and a lid. Let them simmer for 2- 2 ½ hours. The leaves should be tender and easily biteable without any tough chewing. Once done cooking, let them sit in the pot for an extra 20-30 minutes, covered, to absorb any excess water. Flip onto a serving plate, and enjoy.

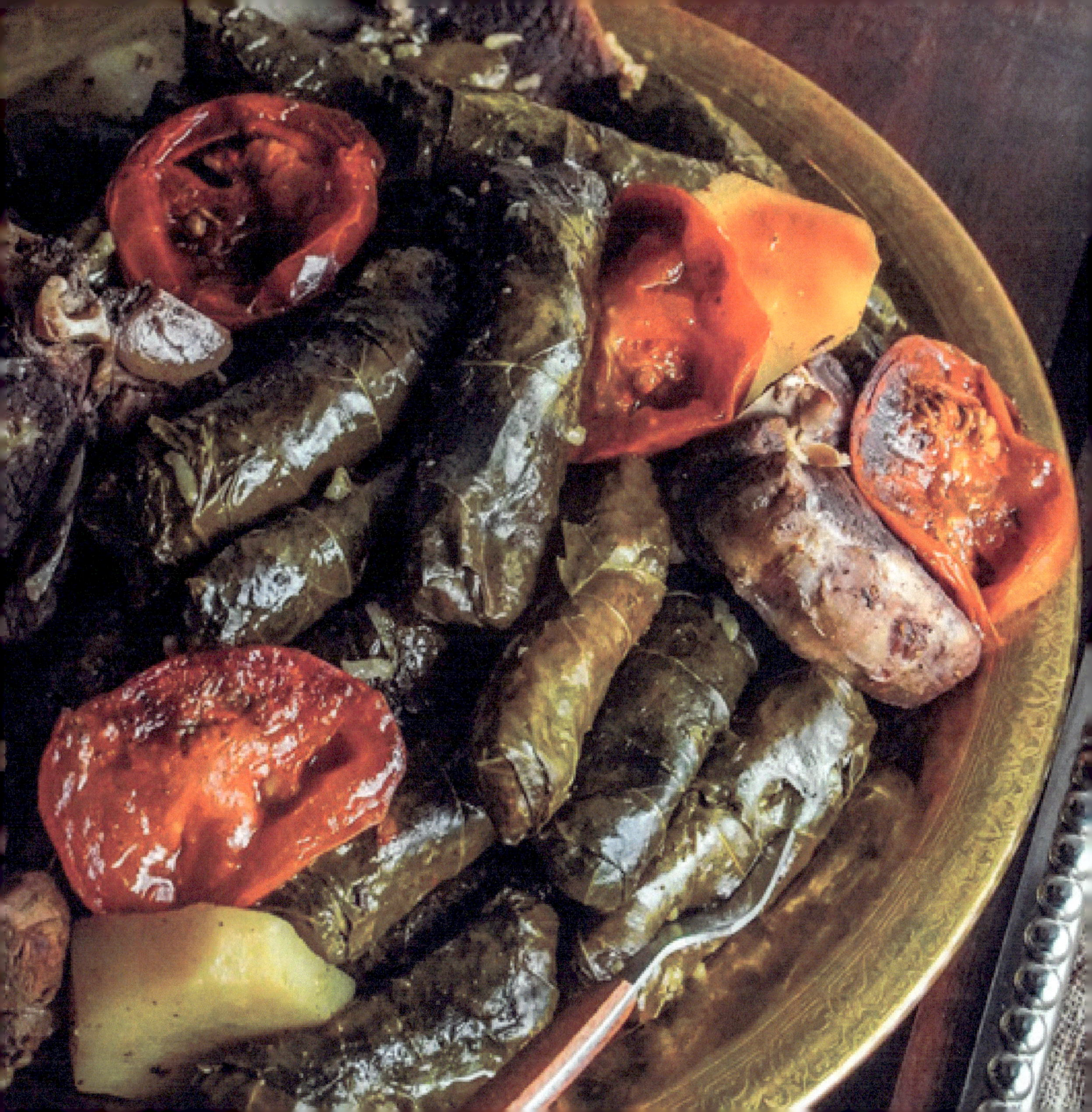

Lamb Qidreh قدرة باللحمة

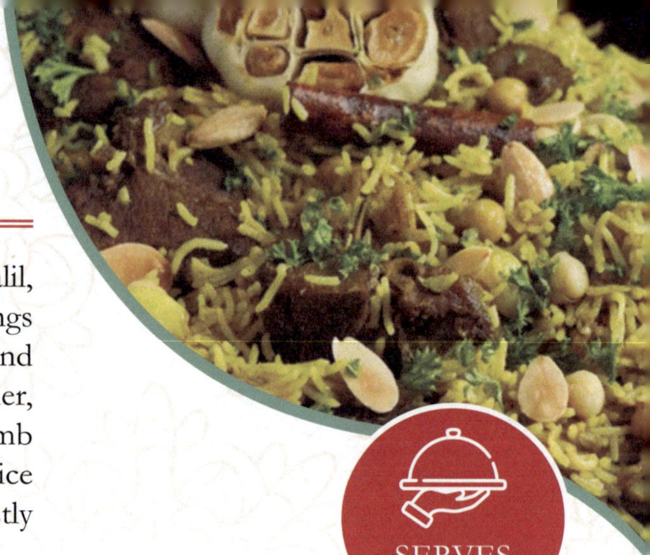

Qidreh is the signature dish of the vibrant city of Al-Khalil, Palestine. It is often made for weddings and celebratory evenings and events. Qidreh is known for its fragrant & garlicky rice and melt-off-the-bone lamb. Traditionally, it is made with lamb shoulder, but oftentimes it is substituted with bone-in chicken, or even lamb shanks. In Al-Khalil, families used to send their lamb and their rice layered in a pot to the butcher to bake in the oven. Now, it is mostly done at home, on the stovetop.

SERVES
4

INGREDIENTS:

For the Lamb & Broth:

- 4 lbs of bone-in lamb shoulder (or loin chops), about 4 large pieces
- 2 tbsp oil
- 1 bay leaf
- 4 cardamom pods
- 1 cinnamon stick
- 1/2 yellow onion
- 4 whole cloves
- 1/2 tsp black pepper
- 1 tbsp 7 spices
- 2 tsp coriander powder
- 1 tsp garlic powder
- 1/2 tsp onion powder
- 1/2 tsp ground cardamom
- 8 garlic cloves
- Water, submerge

The Rice:

- 1 cup basmati, washed and soaked
- 2 tbsp ghee
- 1 tbsp extra virgin olive oil
- 8 garlic cloves,minced
- 4 whole garlic cloves
- 1 small yellow onion, finely chopped
- ⅔ cup canned chickpeas, drained and rinsed
- 1.5 tsp 7 spice
- 1/2 tsp turmeric
- 1 tsp coriander powder
- 1/2 tsp garlic powder
- 1/2 tsp onion powder
- 1/2 tsp cardamom
- 4 cardamom pods
- 1 cinnamon stick
- Salt, to taste

DIRECTIONS:

1. To start, as an optional step, I prefer adding the meat into a large bowl and adding a heaping tsp of salt, and about ½ cup of flour. Then I cover the meat with water and massage the flour into the lamb, and let it sit for half an hour. Thoroughly wash the meat after, and pat dry.I feel that it removes the pungent and gamey smell of the lamb. Feel free to skip this step.
2. Heat up 2 tablespoons of oil in a deep pot on medium-high heat. Add in the lamb pieces and let it heat up for a few minutes. Add the onion half and garlic cloves. Move the meat around gently on all sides. Once a pale grayish-brown color, add the seasonings along with the whole spices. Mix together well and submerged in water. The water needs to be enough to completely cover the lamb, and you may need to add more as it cooks.
3. Let it come to a rolling boil for 6-8 minutes, then cover and lower the heat to medium-low for an hour to an hour and a half, or until the lamb is tender. Once cooked, remove the lamb. Drain and reserve the broth and set aside.
4. As the lamb cooks, wash and soak the basmati rice for 20 minutes, then drain the water.
5. To another pot, add the ghee and olive oil and heat up on medium-high heat.
6. Add the finely chopped onion and saute for a few minutes, until translucent. Now, add in the minced and whole garlic, and drained and rinsed chickpeas. Saute until fragrant and the garlic gets a golden brown color. Add in the drained rice and the seasonings and mix well.
7. Place the lamb pieces directly on top of the rice making sure they're snug.
8. Pour 2 cups of the reserved hot lamb broth. Let it come to a boil for 5 minutes before reducing the heat to medium-low, and covering. Let it simmer for 15-20 minutes, or until the rice is fluffy.
9. Once the rice is done cooking, transfer to a serving tray, and top with toasted almonds and chopped parsley.

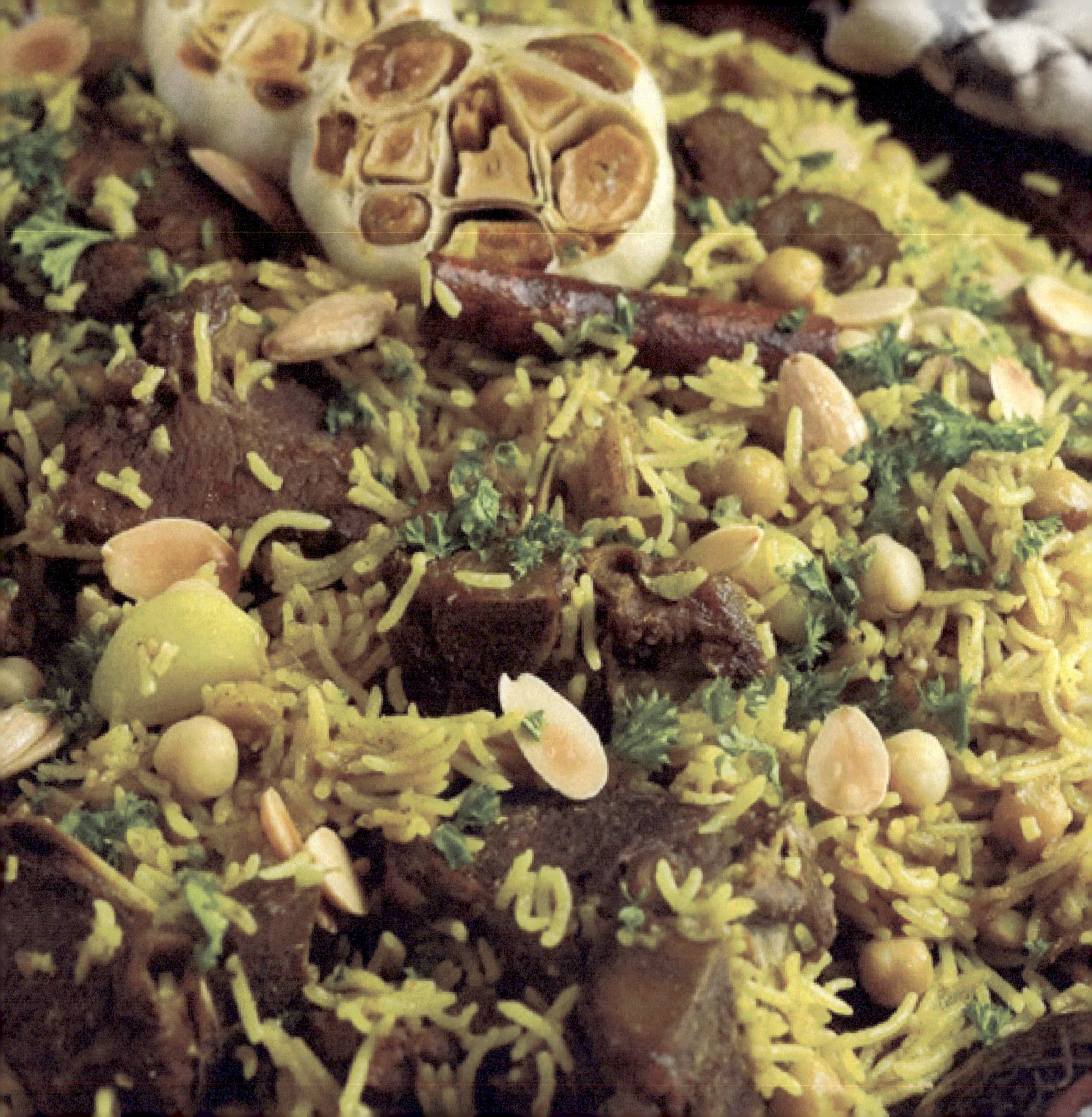

Kufta Bil Bandoura

كفتة بالبندورة

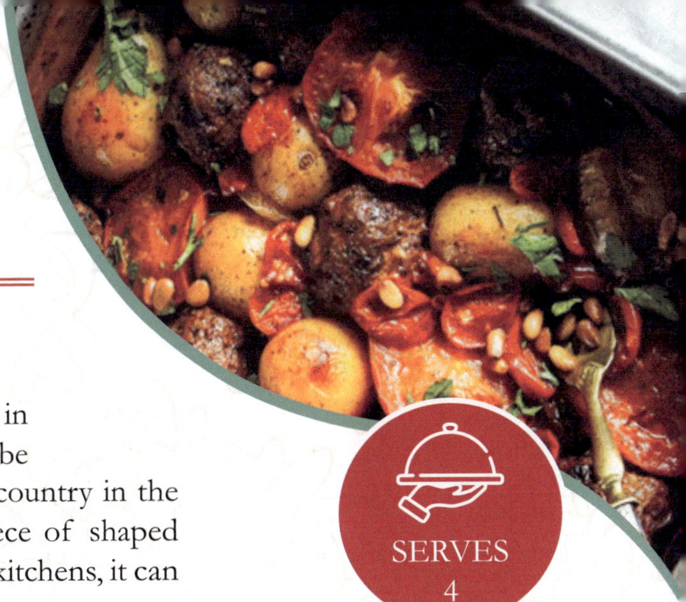

SERVES 4

(Baked Kofta in Tomato Sauce)

Kufta stems from the word that means "ground or beat " in reference to the ground beef or lamb in the dish. It can often be found pronounced as "kefta" or "kofta" depending on which country in the Levant you're in. It is a spiced meatball or small smashed piece of shaped ground beef, often mixed with parsley and onion. In Palestinian kitchens, it can be accompanied by a tomato sauce or a silky tahini sauce.

INGREDIENTS:

- 1 lb 80/20 ground beef or lamb
- ½ bunch parsley
- 6 garlic cloves
- ½ medium yellow onion
- 2 medium roma tomatoes (300g)
- 1 pound baby potatoes, halved (454g)
- ½ tsp 7 spices
- 1 tsp garlic powder
- ½ tsp coriander powder
- ¼ tsp black pepper
- 1 tsp salt
- ½ tsp paprika

Tomato Sauce:

- 2 cups hot water
- 1 15 oz can of tomato sauce (425g)
- 3 tbsp tomato paste
- 1 tbsp pomegranate molasses
- ½ tsp salt
- ¼ tsp black pepper
- 1 tsp dried mint

DIRECTIONS:

1. Preheat the oven to 375.
2. Finely chop the parsley, onion, garlic and tomato. Alternatively, add them to a food processor and pulse until fine. Transfer this mixture to a bowl and add the ground beef. Now, add in the 7 spices, garlic powder, black pepper, salt, and paprika. Mix well.

3. Shape the meatballs in 1 ½ - 2 inch balls. Set aside. Wash and cut the potatoes, then pat dry. If you're using larger potatoes, peel them too. Fry or air fry the potatoes until golden. Transfer the potatoes and the meatballs into a deep baking dish.
4. To make the sauce, mix together the tomato sauce, water, and tomato paste. Mix together well until tomato paste is dissolved. Add the pomegranate molasses, salt, black pepper, and dried mint. Mix until well combined.
5. Pour the sauce over the meatballs and potatoes and cover with aluminum foil. Bake at 375 for 25-35 minutes, or until the beef reaches an internal temperature of 160 degrees.
6. Serve with pita bread.

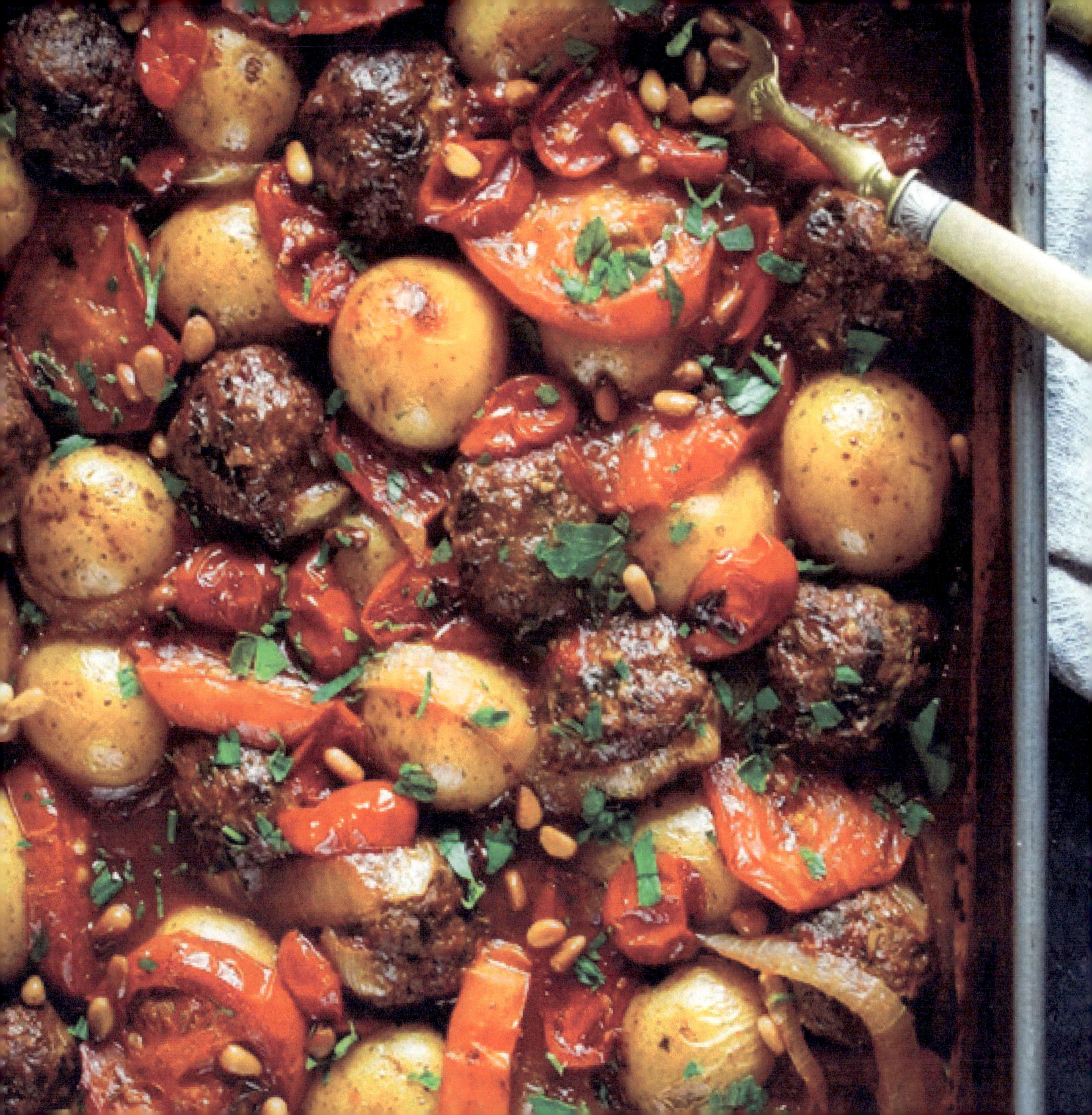

Macarona Bil Lahme

معكرونة باللحمة

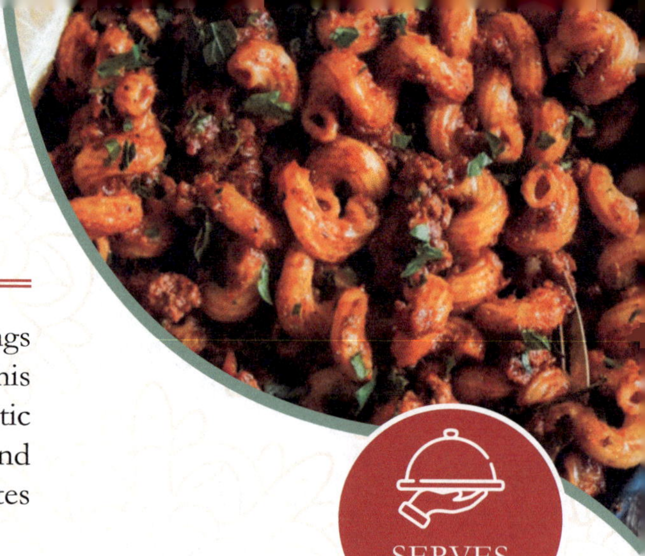

SERVES
3-4

Macarona Bil lahme is a hearty and flavorful dish that brings together the best of Middle Eastern and Italian influences. This fusion creation marries savory ground beef cooked in aromatic spices, leading to a rich and satisfying sauce that coats every strand of pasta. The result is a delicious harmony of textures and tastes that will transport you to your childhood.

INGREDIENTS:

- 12 oz elbow pasta
- 1 lb 80/20% lean ground beef
- 1 medium yellow onion, finely chopped
- 2 tbsp oil
- 3 garlic cloves, minced
- 30 oz tomato sauce
- 2 tbsp tomato paste
- 1 ½ tsp7 spices
- 1 tsp coriander powder
- 1 tsp garlic powder
- 1 tsp onion powder
- ½ tsp ground cumin
- ½ tsp black pepper
- Salt, to taste

DIRECTIONS:

1. Begin by cooking our pasta according to package instructions.
2. Add a medium-sized pot to the stove on medium-high heat. Add the oil.
3. Toss in the finely chopped onion and saute until translucent, about 3-5 minutes.
4. Add in the minced garlic and saute until fragrant, another 1-2 minutes.
5. Now, add in the ground beef and break it up as much as possible. You do not want overly large chunks of beef.
6. Brown the beef well, making sure it is thoroughly cooked.
7. Sprinkle in the seasonings and mix well.

8. Add the tomato paste along with the tomato sauce and mix well. Cover and let the beef cook in the sauce for 6-8 minutes on medium heat.
9. Once the sauce has simmered, add in the drained pasta. Mix well to combine and serve.
10. Garnish with toasted nuts or chopped parsley.

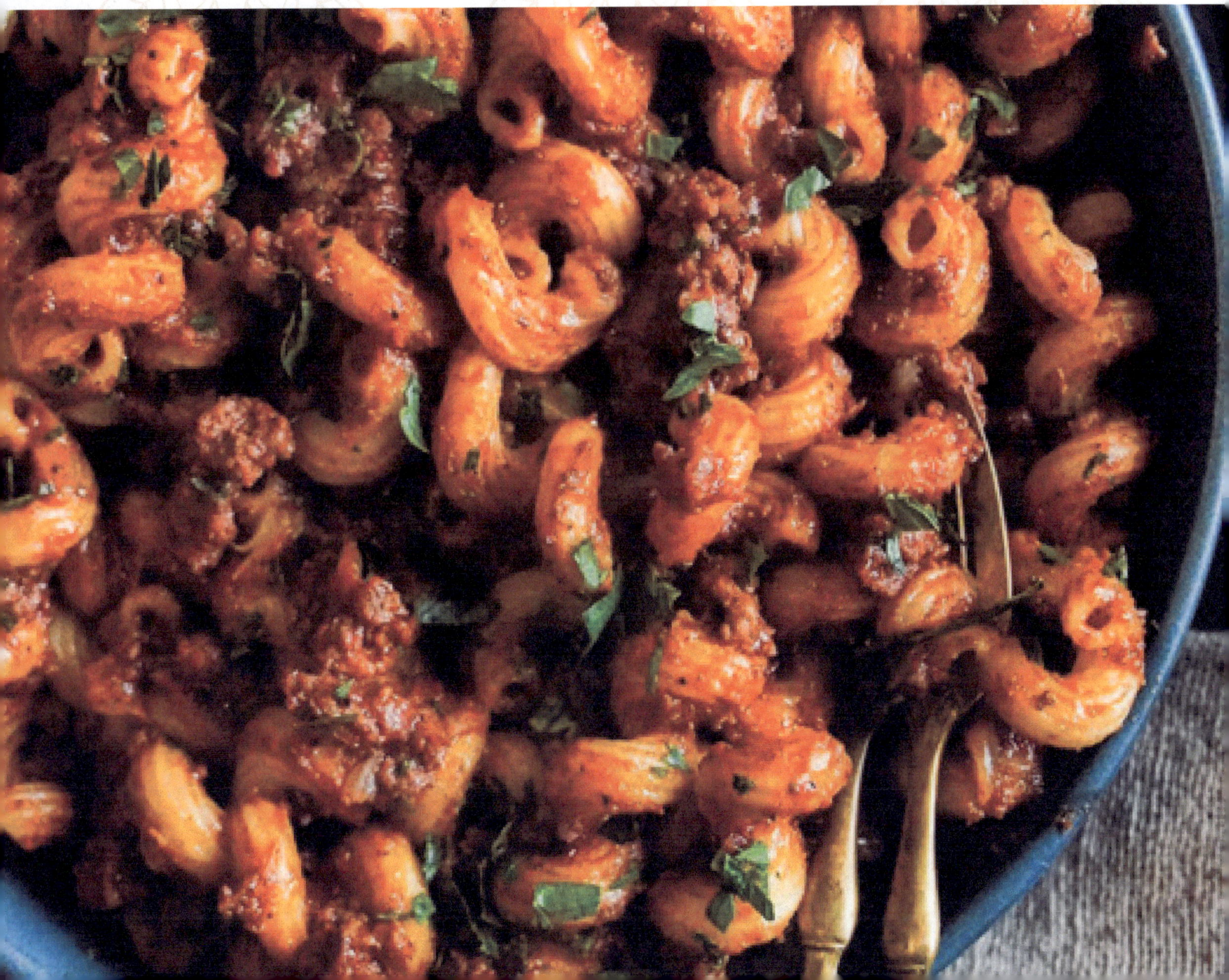

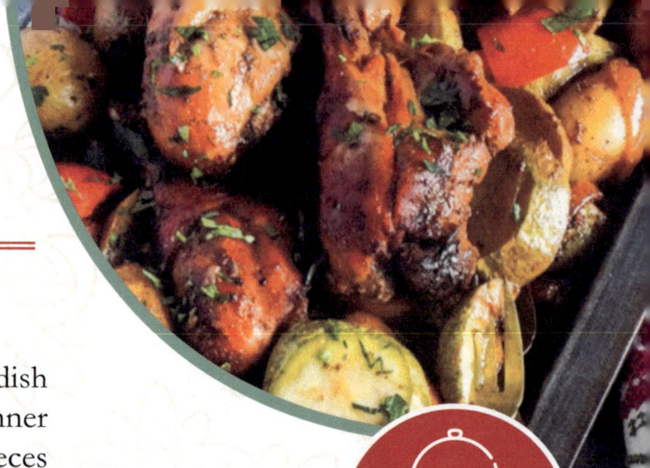

Jaj Ou Khodar صينية دجاج وخضار

(Chicken and Vegetable Bake)

This Middle Eastern Chicken Bake is a flavorful and aromatic dish that brings the rich and diverse spices of the Middle East to the dinner table. This hearty bake typically features succulent chicken pieces marinated in a blend of spices such as sumac, coriander, turmeric, and paprika, creating a harmonious fusion of leveled flavors.

SERVES 4-6

The chicken is often paired with vegetables like bell peppers, onions, and potatoes, adding freshness,depth of flavor, and vibrant colors to the dish. The use of garlic, lemon, and olive oil contributes to the robust and savory profile, enhancing the overall taste experience.

INGREDIENTS:

- 8 bone-in chicken thighs or drumsticks
- ⅓ cup plain whole milk yogurt
- ¼ cup extra virgin olive oil
- 1 tbsp lemon juice
- 3 garlic cloves, minced
- 2 tsp 7 spices
- ½ tbsp paprika
- ½ tbsp sumac
- ½ tsp black pepper
- ½ tbsp salt, or to taste
- ½ tbsp garlic powder
- ½ tsp turmeric

Vegetables:

- ½ lb baby potatoes, halved
- 2 medium zucchini squash, cut into approximately ½ inch thick rounds
- 1 cup baby carrots
- ½ a large red onion, cut into 1 inch squares
- 1 red bell pepper, cut into squares or thin slices

DIRECTIONS:

1. Preheat oven to 400 F
2. In a bowl, combine together the whole milk yogurt, the extra virgin olive oil, lemon juice, and minced garlic.

3. Add in the chicken pieces and combine well to coat. You can let this marinate or use right away.
4. In a separate small bowl, combine together the salt, black pepper, sumac, paprika, garlic powder, turmeric, and 7 spices. Mix well.
5. Line a 9x13 inch pan with parchment paper. Add the coated chicken.
6. Add the cut-up vegetable pieces, layering them around the chicken evenly. Make sure each chicken piece is not overlapping on another.
7. Sprinkle the seasoning mix all over the chicken, and mix well using clean hands. Cover with aluminum foil.
8. Bake at 400 F for 40-55 minutes, or until the chicken reaches an internal temperature of 165 F.
9. Serve with rice, salad, or pita bread.

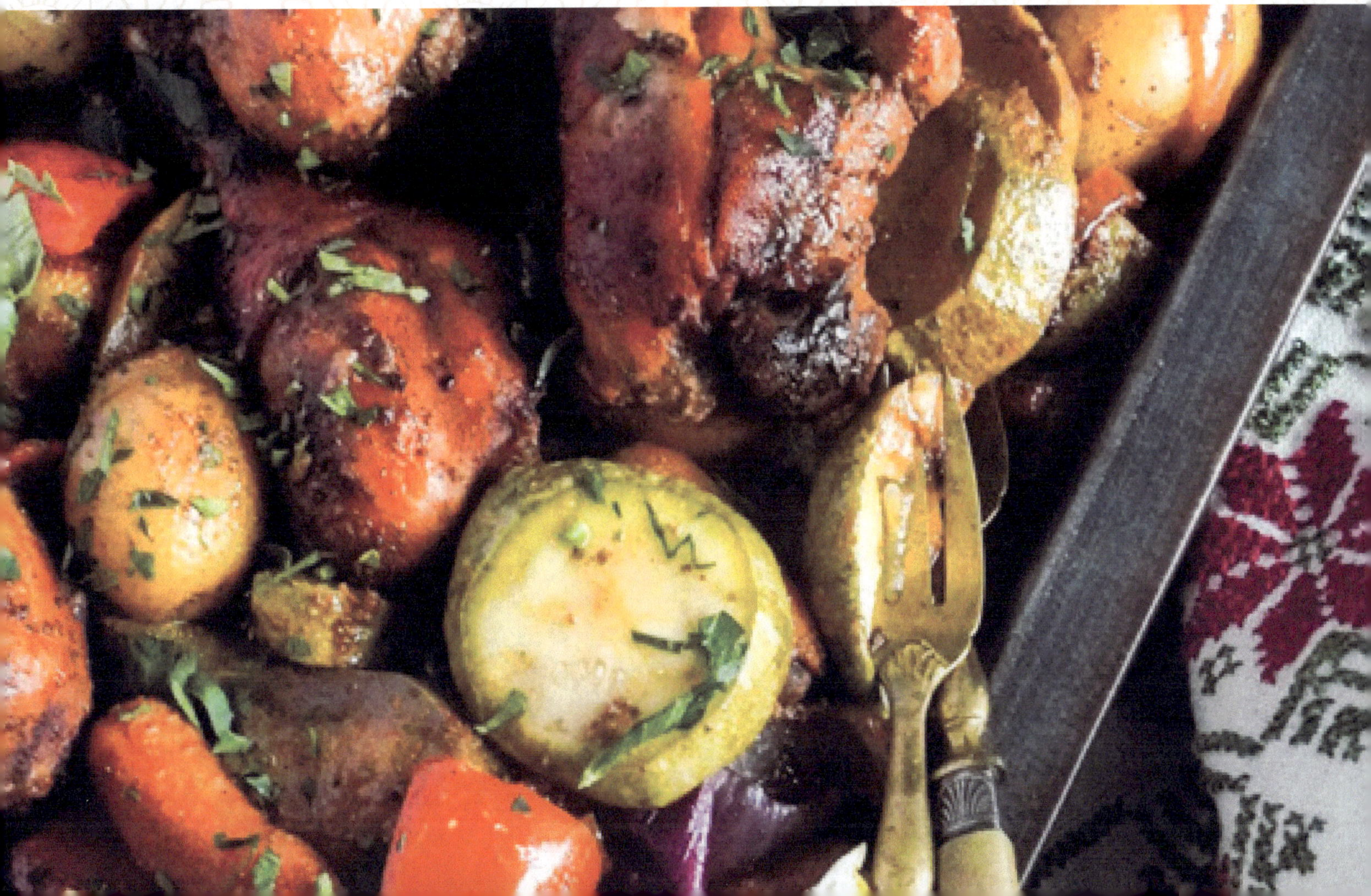

Quick Chicken Shawarma

شاورما دجاج

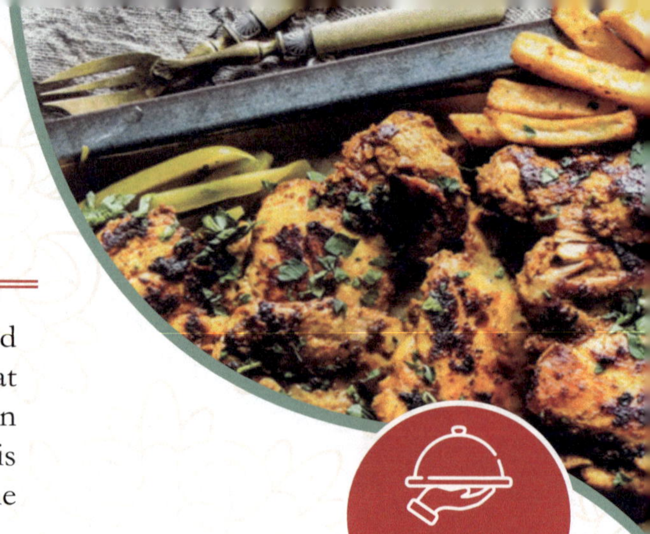

Tender, grilled chicken pieces infused with aromatic spices and marinated to perfection in a delectable yogurt marinade that make the flavor traditional yet mouth-watering, this chicken shawarma recipe will be in your dinner rotations for a while! This is the quicker take on my most popular shawarma recipe on the Falasteenifoodie blog.

INGREDIENTS:

- 2 ½ lbs boneless skinless chicken thighs
- ⅓ cup plain whole milk yogurt
- 3 tbsp extra virgin olive oil
- 2 tbsp lemon juice
- 4 garlic cloves, minced
- 1 tbsp 7 spices
- 1 ½ tsp paprika
- 1 ½ tsp garlic powder
- 1 tsp onion powder
- 1 tsp salt
- ¼ tsp black pepper
- ½ tsp turmeric
- ¼ tsp Aleppo pepper

To Serve:

- Middle Eastern pickled cucumbers
- Middle Eastern pickled turnips
- Toum (garlic sauce)
- Fries
- Shrak bread (Markouk) or flour tortilla

DIRECTIONS:

1. To speed up the marinating process, take each chicken thigh and pierce it lightly with a fork a few times in multiple spots.
2. Add the chicken thighs to a bowl.
3. Combine the minced garlic, yogurt, olive oil, and lemon juice. Add to the chicken.
4. Add all the spices and mix well. Cover and let it sit until you preheat your pan and prepare your toppings.
5. Preheat a pan on medium heat. Let it get hot.

6. Lightly grease your pan, with oil or cooking spray.
7. Add your chicken thighs a few at a time making sure to not overcrowd the pan.
8. Let each side cook for about 5-6 minutes before attempting to flip.
9. Once flipped, cook for an additional 6-8 minutes, or until the internal temperature reaches 165 F and the chicken is no longer pink.
10. Once cooked, transfer to a plate and immediately cover. Let it rest for 5 minutes before slicing into thin strips.
11. Serve on shrak bread or tortilla, with garlic sauce, fries, and an assortment of Middle Eastern pickles. You could also wrap the sandwich and press it to make it crispy.

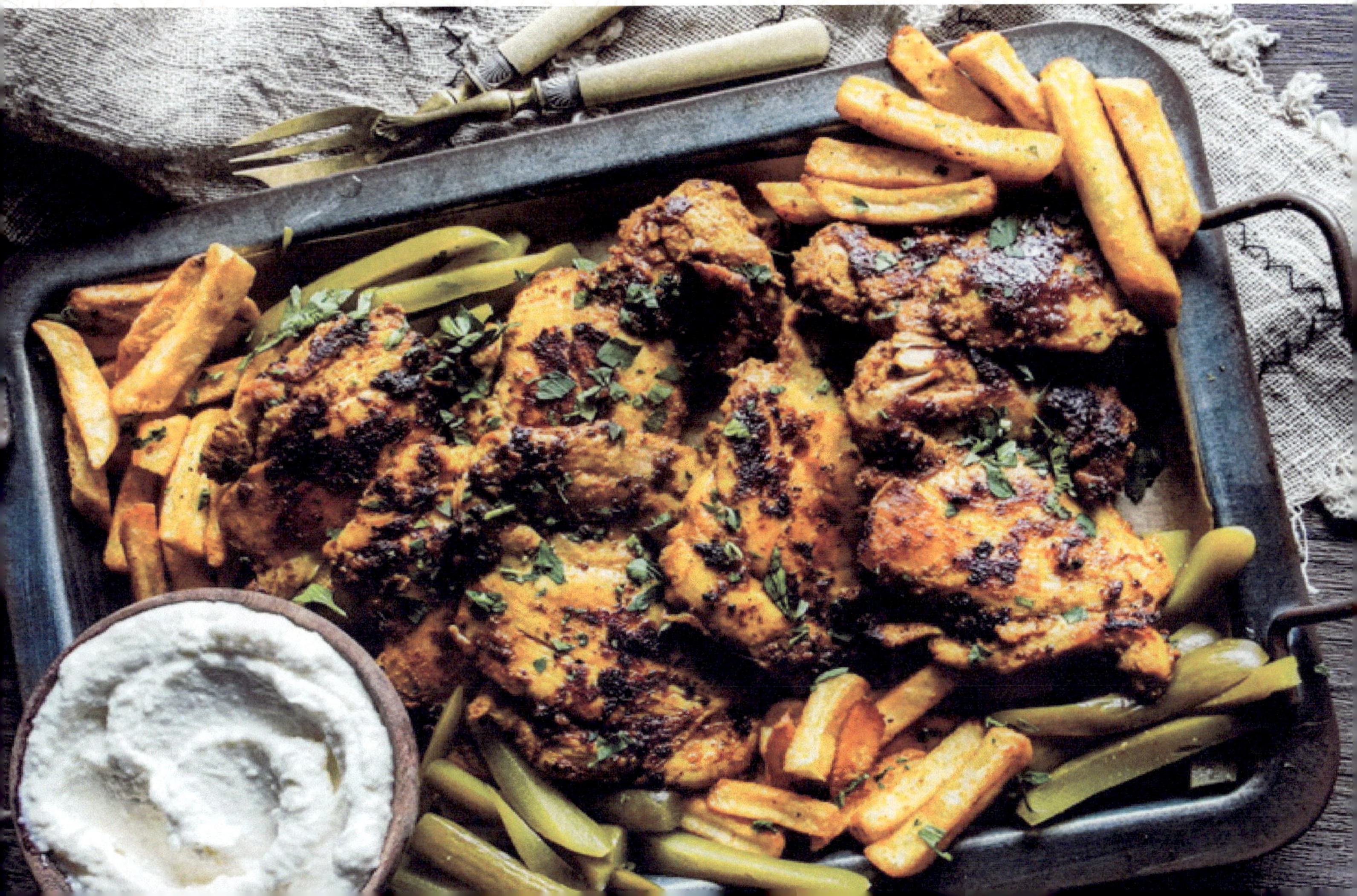

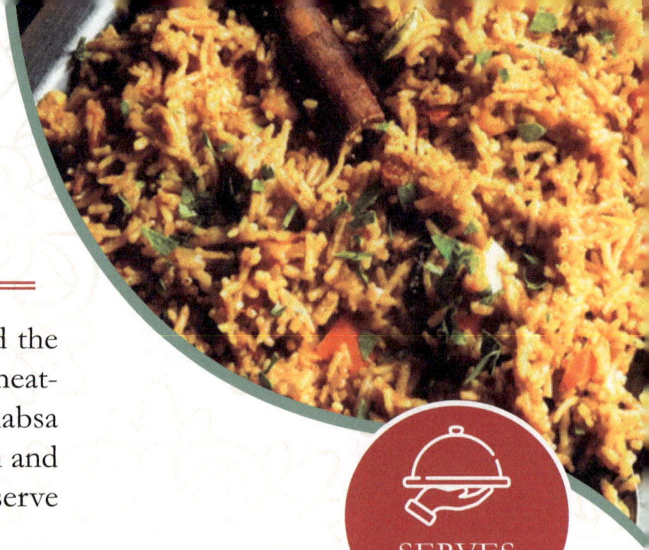

Vegetarian Kabsa Rice

ارز الكبسة

Kabsa is a traditional and flavorful dish that is often considered the national dish of Saudi Arabia. It is a spiced rice dish with meat- typically lamb, chicken, or beef- and a blend of aromatic spices. Kabsa is popular across the Arabian Peninsula and is known for its rich and fragrant flavor profile. Oftentimes, I make the rice on its own to serve as a vegetarian dish, or to serve with a baked leg of lamb.

SERVES 4

INGREDIENTS:

- 2 cups basmati rice, washed and soaked
- 3 tbsp avocado or canola oil
- 1½ large yellow onions, finely chopped
- 6 garlic cloves, finely minced
- ½ inch knob of ginger, finely chopped
- 1 roma tomato, finely chopped
- 1 bell pepper, finely chopped
- Jalapenos, to taste
- 1 dry lemon
- 1 cinnamon stick
- 3 cardamom pods
- 2 whole cloves
- 2 tsp salt, or to taste
- 1 tbsp kabsa spices (see below)
- 1½ tbsp tomato paste
- 4 cups hot water

Kabsa Spice Mix:

- ½ tsp cinnamon
- ½ tsp black pepper
- 1 tsp garlic powder
- 1 tsp onion powder
- 1 tsp curry powder
- ½ tsp turmeric
- ½ tsp ground cardamom
- 1 ½ tsp 7 spices
- 1 tsp coriander powder

DIRECTIONS:

1. Wash and soak the rice in room temperature water for 20 minutes. Drain and set aside.

2. In a pot on medium-high heat, add the oil. Let it heat up before adding in the finely chopped onion.
3. Saute for 2-3 minutes, then add the minced garlic, finely chopped ginger, and bell pepper. If you're using jalapenos, add as well.
4. Add the whole spices; such as the cardamom pods, cinnamon stick, whole cloves, and dried lemon (loomi). Saute everything together for another few minutes, until the vegetables are softened and the onions and garlic turn a golden brown color.
5. Add in the finely chopped tomatoes. Let them cook for about 2-3 minutes, or until softened.
6. Add in the drained rice, and mix.
7. Add in the ground kabsa seasonings, and the salt. Mix.
8. Mix the tomato paste with the 4 cups of hot water until dissolved. Pour over the rice.
9. Let the mixture come to a boil. Let it boil for about 3-5 minutes, or until the liquid begins touching the surface of the rice. Immediately lower the heat to low, and cover.
10. Let it cook on low for 15-20 minutes, or until the rice is fluffy.
11. Once done, transfer to a serving platter and top with toasted sliced almonds and chopped parsley.

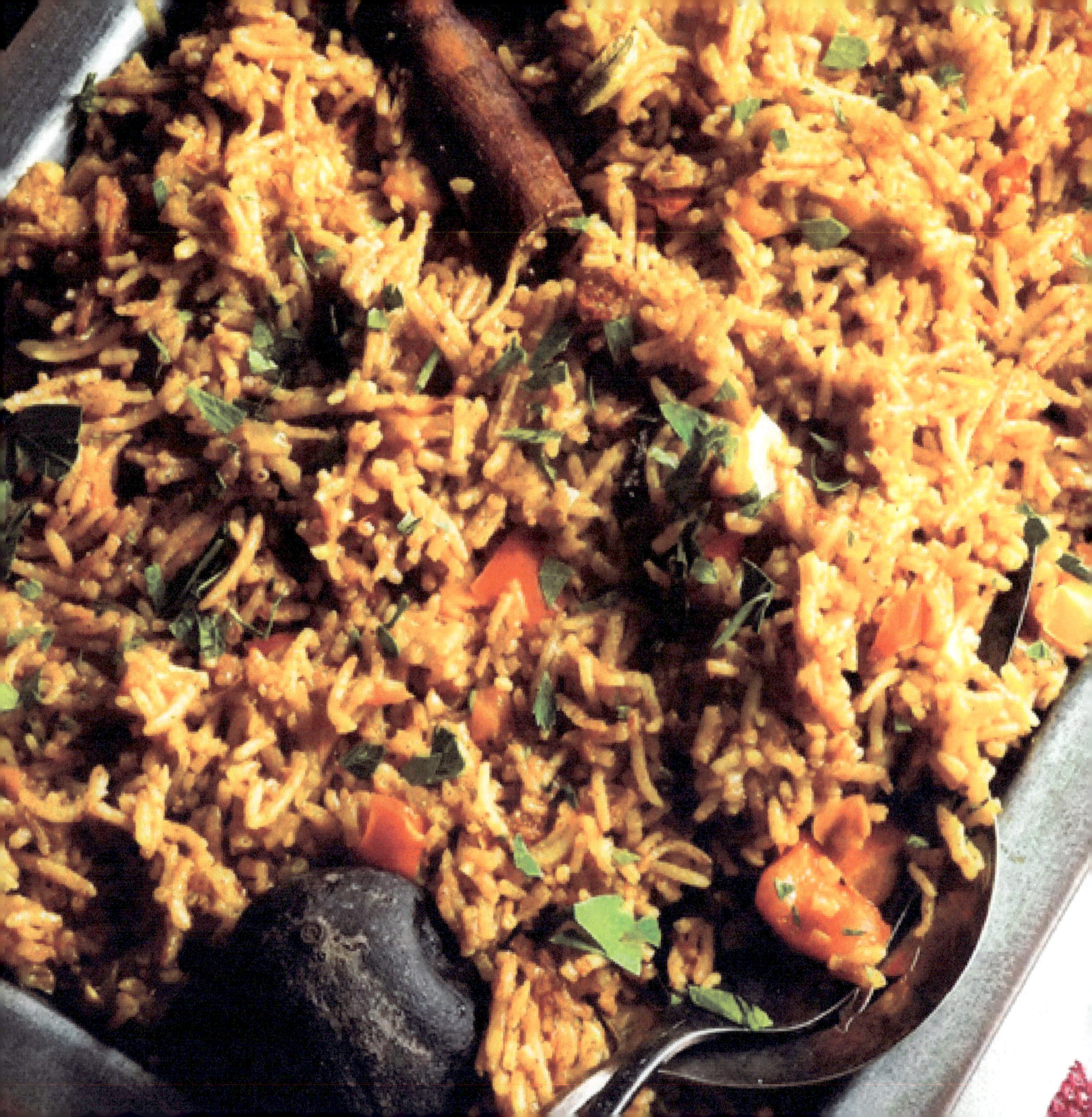

Sayadieh صيادية

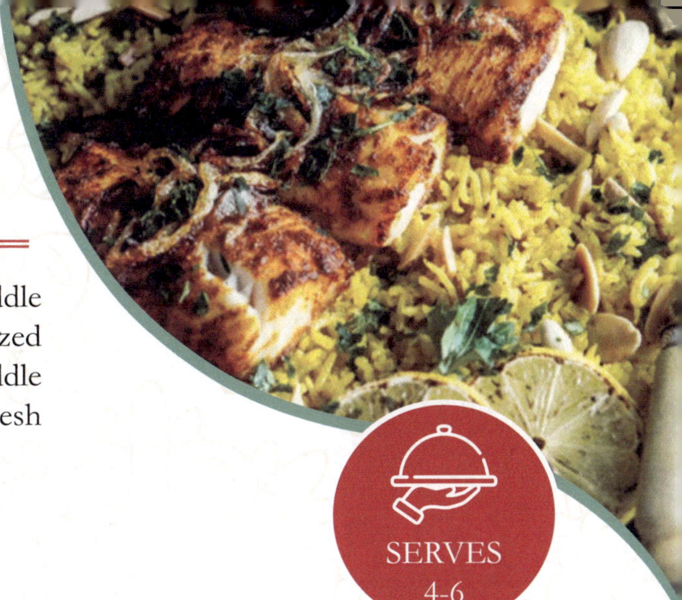

Sayadieh, also spelled Sayadiya or Sayadiah, is a traditional Middle Eastern dish that features seasoned rice, fish, and a rich caramelized onion topping. This flavorful and aromatic dish is popular in Middle Eastern cuisine, particularly along the coastal regions where fresh seafood is readily available.

SERVES 4-6

INGREDIENTS:

The Fish:

- 6 white fish filets pieces, such as tilapia
- 3 tbsp extra virgin olive oil
- 1 tsp paprika
- 1 tsp cumin
- ½ tsp black pepper
- 2 tsp 7 spices
- 2 tsp coriander powder
- 1 tsp garlic powder
- 1 ½ tsp salt, or to taste

The Rice:

- 2 cups basmati rice, washed and soaked
- 1 medium yellow onion, finely chopped
- 3 cloves garlic, minced
- ½ a red bell pepper
- 2 tbsp neutral oil, such as canola or avocado oil
- 2 tsp salt, or to taste
- ¾ tsp turmeric
- 2 tsp 7 spices
- 2 tsp coriander powder
- ½ tsp ground cardamom
- 4 cups of hot water

To serve:

- Toasted almond slivers
- Caramelized onions
- Lemon wedges

DIRECTIONS:

1. Preheat the oven to 350 F.
2. Start by washing the rice, and soaking it for 20 minutes. Drain and set aside.
3. To prepare the fish, mix the extra virgin olive oil with the paprika, cumin, chili powder, garlic powder, salt, black pepper, and 7 spices. Brush on top of the fish pieces on both sides.

4. Place the fish pieces on a baking sheet lined with parchment paper. Bake at 350 F for 15-20 minutes, or until the fish flakes with a fork.
5. To make the rice, add the oil to a pot on medium-high heat.
6. Add in the finely chopped onion, bell pepper, and the minced garlic. Saute for 5-6 minutes or until fragrant.
7. Add the previously washed and soaked rice. Add in the remaining seasonings and mix together well.
8. Add 4 cups of hot water and stir. Let it come to a boil, and let it continue boiling for 2-3 minutes before covering and reducing the heat to low. Let it simmer on low for 15-20 minutes, or until the rice is fluffy and has absorbed all the water.
9. To serve, add the fish on top of the rice. Garnish with caramelized onions, toasted slivered almonds, and lemon wedges.

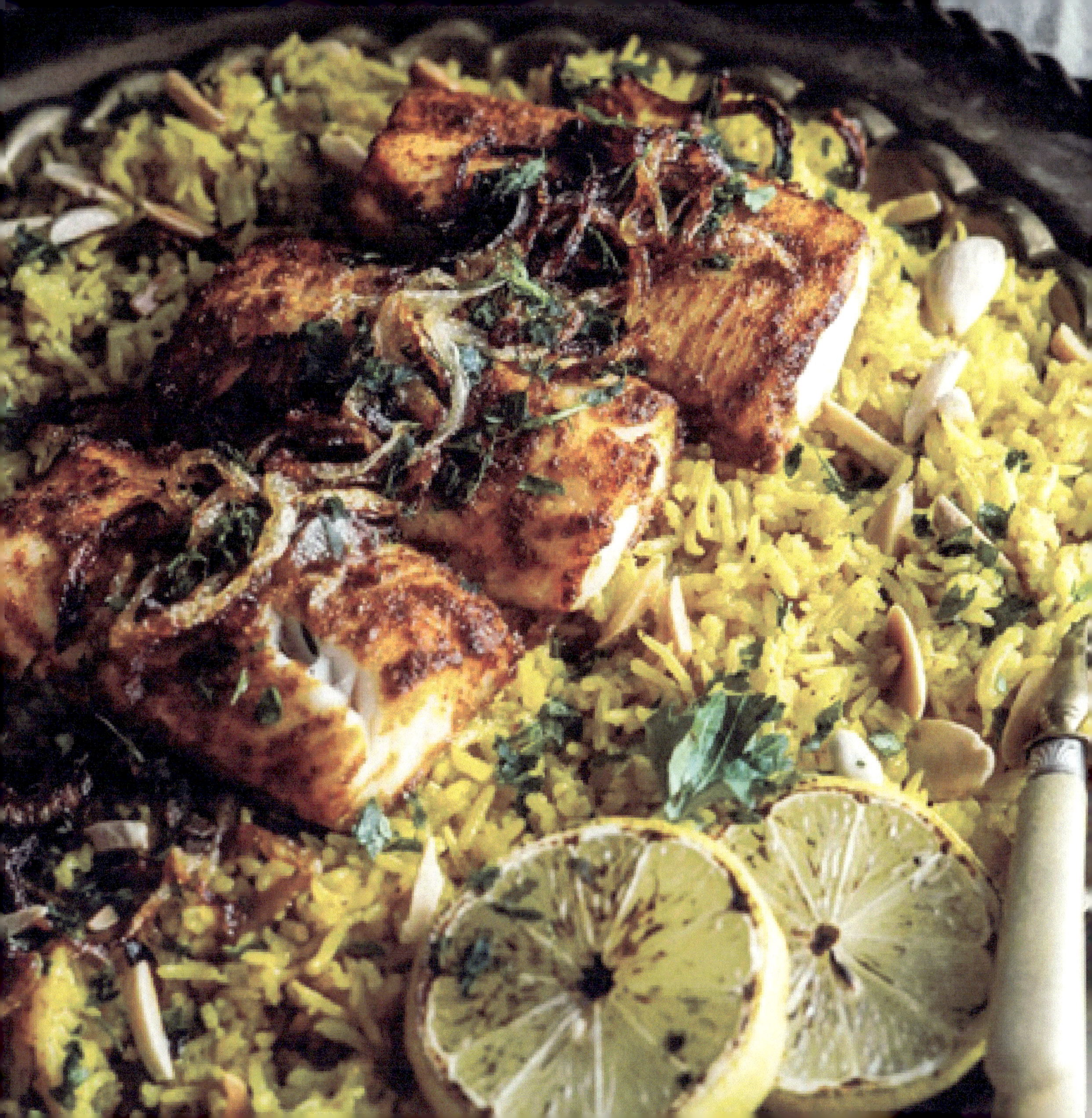

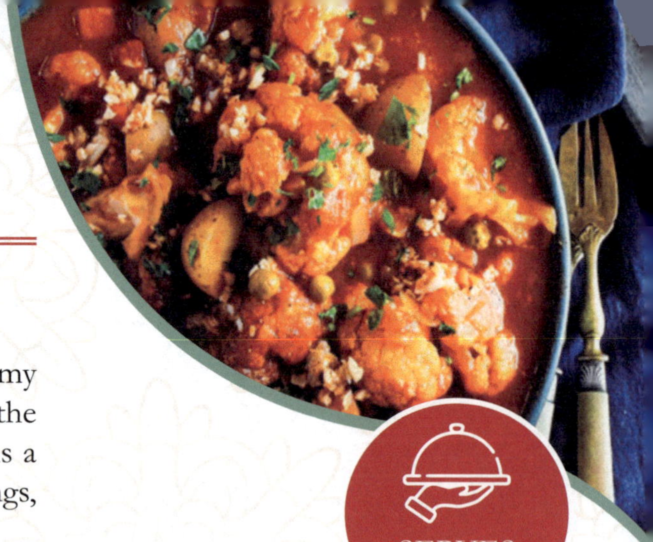

Yakhnet Khoudar يخنة خضار

(Vegetable Stew)

Growing up, in an attempt to make us eat more vegetables, my mom made us a stew very similar to this. It would be filled to the brim with soft and braised eye-catching vegetables. The result is a delicious stew warmed with common Arab spices and seasonings, and leaves you with the feeling of ultimate comfort.

SERVES 3-4

INGREDIENTS:

- 1 medium yellow onion, finely chopped
- 3 garlic cloves, minced
- ½ lb baby potatoes, cubed
- 1 lb cauliflower florets, air fried, baked, or deep fried
- 1 cup frozen carrots & peas
- 3 cups water
- 1 15 oz can tomato sauce
- 2 tbsp tomato paste
- 2 tbsp neutral oil

Seasonings:

- 2 tsp 7 spices
- ½ tsp salt
- ¼ tsp black pepper
- 1 tsp coriander powder
- 1 tsp garlic powder
- ½ tsp turmeric

Tassha(Garlic topping):

- 6 garlic cloves, minced
- 1 tbsp oil or butter

DIRECTIONS:

1. Cut the cauliflower into florets and fry or air fry until golden. You can also air fry or bake the potatoes.
2. Heat the pot on high heat. Add the finely chopped onions and garlic. Saute until golden brown.
3. Add the cooked cauliflower, potatoes, and the peas and carrots. Mix well and let them cook for 3-5 minutes, stirring occasionally.
4. Add the 7 spices, salt, black pepper, coriander powder, garlic powder, and turmeric. Mix well.
5. Mix the tomato paste with 3 cups of hot water. Add to the vegetables, along with the tomato sauce. Mix everything until well combined. Let this cook on medium low heat for 20-25 minutes, or until the potatoes are fork tender.

6. In a small pan, heat 1 tbsp of oil on high heat. Add the 6 minced garlic cloves and saute until golden. Pour this mixture (tassha) on top of the vegetable stew. Stir well.
7. Serve with some white rice, vermicelli rice, or pita bread.

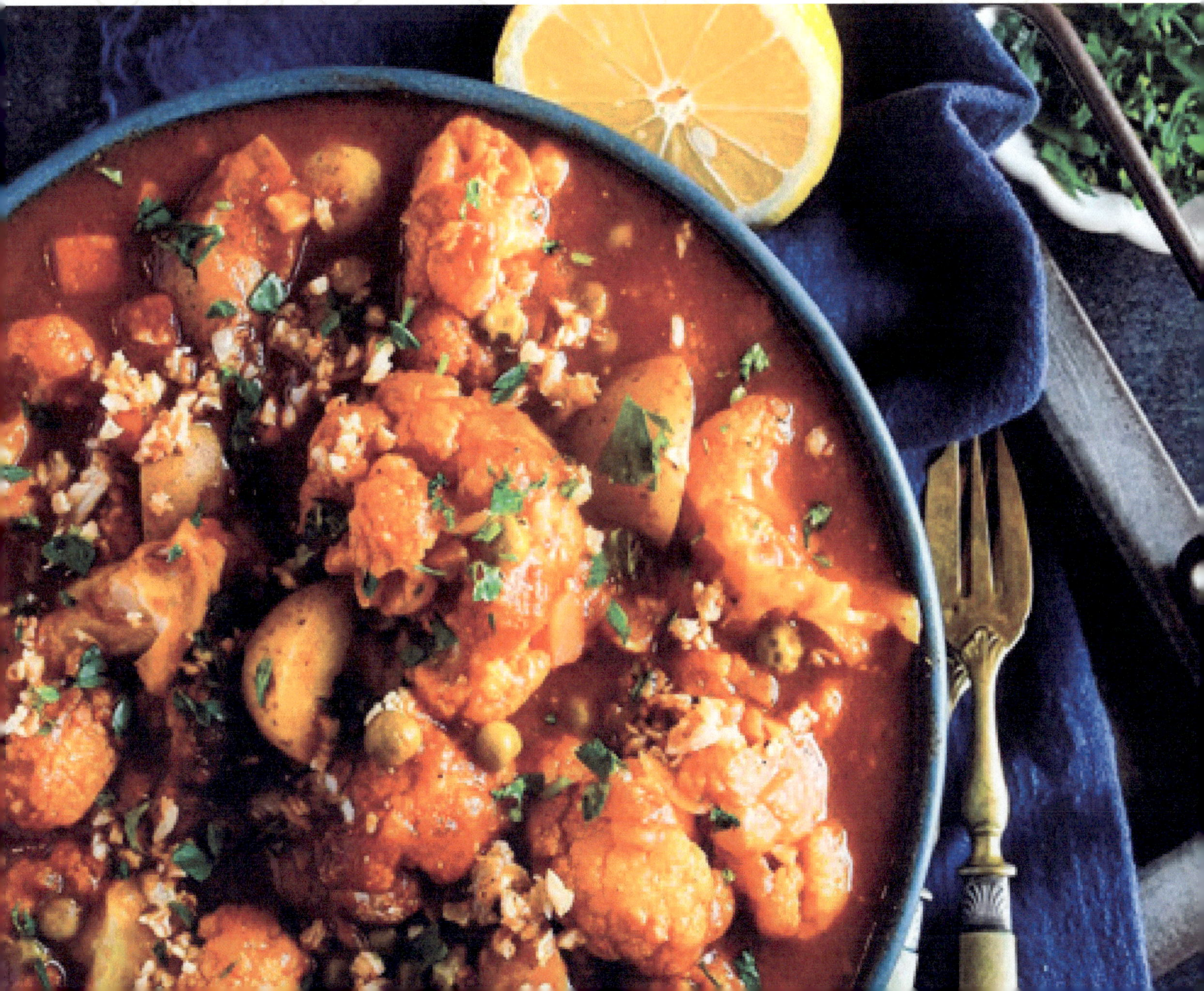

Arab Essentials

أساسيات عربية

These are the essentials to have in your fridge, pantry or freezer. From za'atar to dessert fillings.

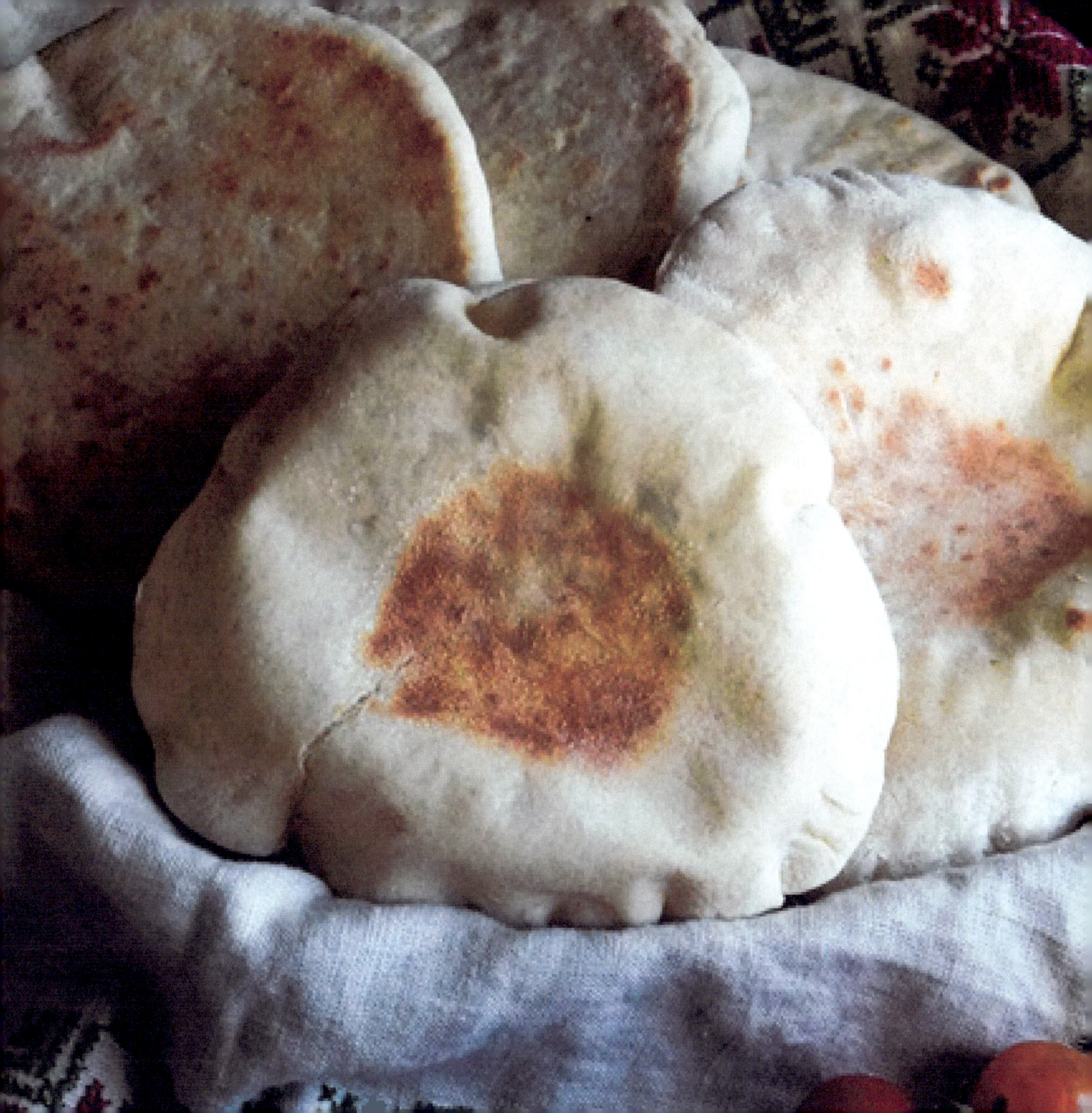

10 Minute Dough عجينة العشر دقائق

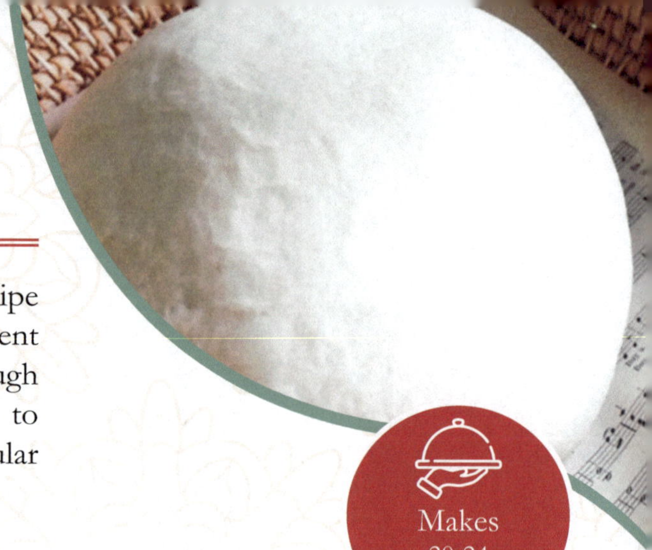

Makes 20-24 dough balls

"Ten-minute dough" typically refers to a quick and easy dough recipe that can be prepared in about ten minutes, making it a convenient option for various baked goods. It is an extremely popular dough recipe in the Middle East because it allows for larger batches to be prepared quickly. This recipe is also one of the most popular recipes on the Falasteenifoodie blog.

INGREDIENTS:

- 5 cups all-purpose flour
- ½ cup oil, could be vegetable oil,canola oil, or olive oil
- 1 tbsp active dry yeast
- 1-2 tbsp granulated sugar, or ¼ cup for sweeter doughs
- 3 tbsp powdered milk (optional)
- 1 tsp salt
- 2 cups warm water or warm whole milk
- 1 tsp baking powder

DIRECTIONS:

1. In a large bowl, start by mixing 2 cups of all-purpose flour, the active dry yeast, the granulated sugar, the baking powder, powdered milk (if you're using it), and the salt. Then, add the warm water or whole milk.
2. Mix them all together until it's smooth using your hands or a stand mixer. It'll be liquidly, but that's fine. Cover it, and let it sit in a warm place for 10-15 minutes until it becomes bubbly. You can cover it with a blanket or two.
3. Once the 10 minutes are over, add the remaining 3 cups of all-purpose flour and the oil to the dough. Mix them well.
4. Knead it for about 5-10 minutes. It will come together really quickly.
5. Now, it's ready to use for anything your family asks for. Some closed pastries might need an egg wash.

Pro Tips:

» If you choose to use or not use powdered milk, the amount of liquid (2 cups) does NOT change.

» For sweeter doughs, such as cinnamon rolls, add more sugar to the dough.

» The water or milk you use should be warm. You can test it with your fingertip. If it is too hot, it will kill the yeast and your dough will not rise. If it is cold, the yeast will take longer to activate and your dough will need a longer time to rise.

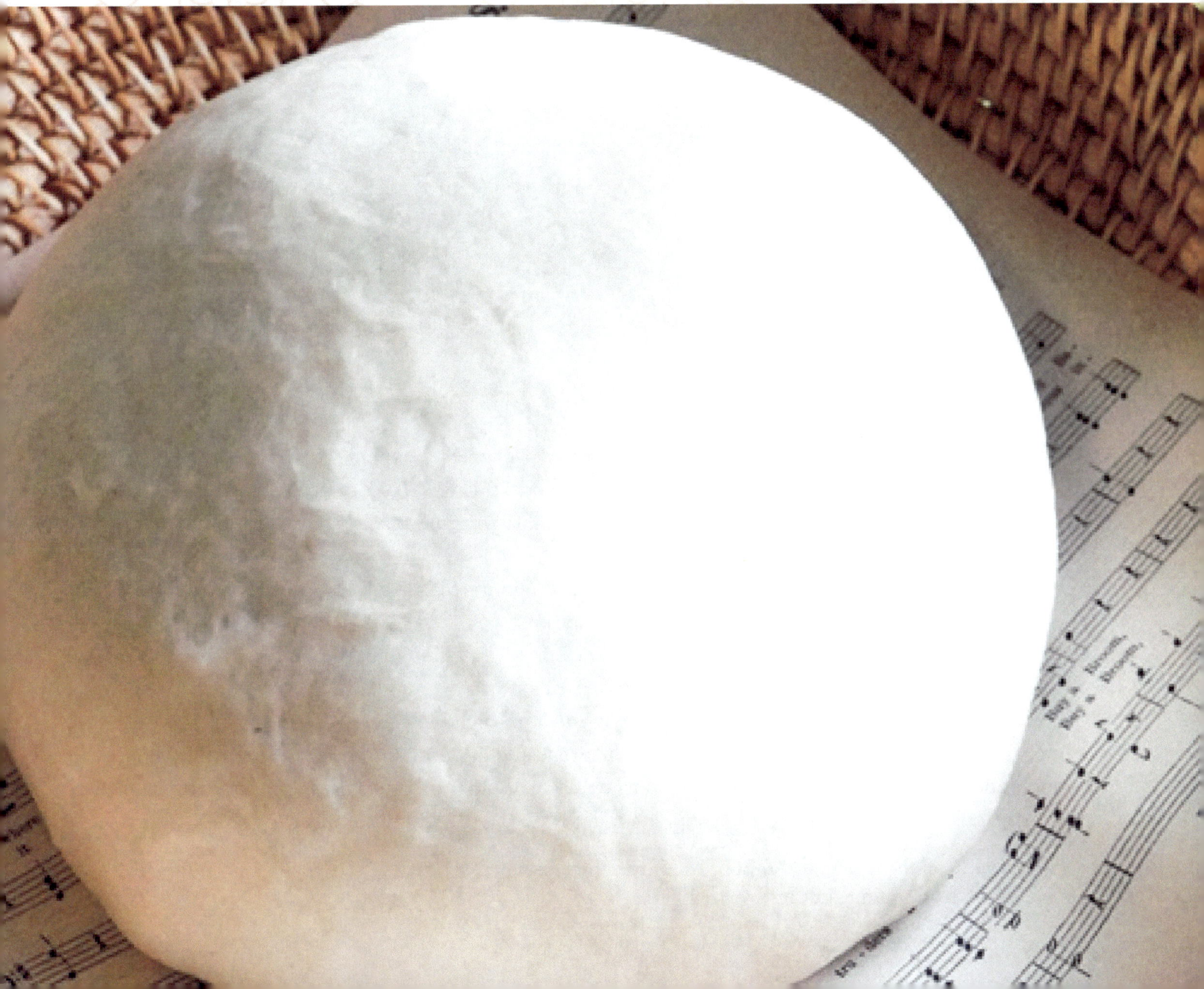

Pita Bread (Kmaaj) خبز كماج

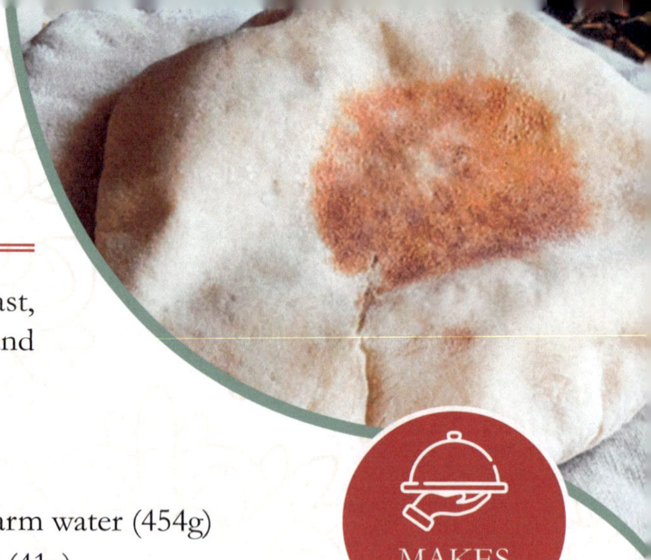

A Middle Eastern household staple. These are eaten for breakfast, lunch, dinner, or even as part of a snack. These are so good and they keep in the freezer really well!

MAKES 12-14

INGREDIENTS:

- 4 and a 1/2 cups bread flour (540g)
- 2 tsp active dry yeast (6g)
- 2 tsp granulated sugar (6g)
- 2 cups warm water (454g)
- 3 tbsp oil (41g)
- 2 tsp salt (6g)

DIRECTIONS:

1. Add the yeast, sugar, and 1 cup water to a bowl. Mix well and let it activate until frothy. This should take about 10 minutes.
2. Add the flour and salt and mix with a wooden spoon until a scraggly dough comes together, then transfer to a stand mixer.
3. Using the dough hook, and on medium speed, drizzle in 2 tablespoons of oil, and the remaining water. Scrape down the sides if needed and let the machine knead it for 10-15 minutes. The dough might be sticky, but form it into a ball and transfer to a clean bowl. Cover, and place in a warm spot to let it double in size, about 1-2 hours.
4. Once doubled, flour your surface well and divide the dough into 12-14 pieces. Cover loosely with a clean kitchen towel, and let them rise for another 15 minutes.
5. Once rested, flour a clean surface well once again and spread each dough ball into a 5-6 inch circle, making sure the thickness is even all round. Let it rest for 15 mins.
6. Meanwhile, heat up a pan (cast iron preferably) on medium-high heat and make sure it's hot.
7. Once the dough circles have rested, add one to the preheated pan and wait to see a sign of bubbling. Once bubbles occur, flip and let the magic work on its own. It should puff on its own. Once puffy, flip again to get some color before removing and wrapping in a towel to not dry out before storing.

Pro Tip: If you roll the dough too thin or roll it too thick, it will not puff up and create a pocket. The dough needs plenty of resting time, but it's worth it.

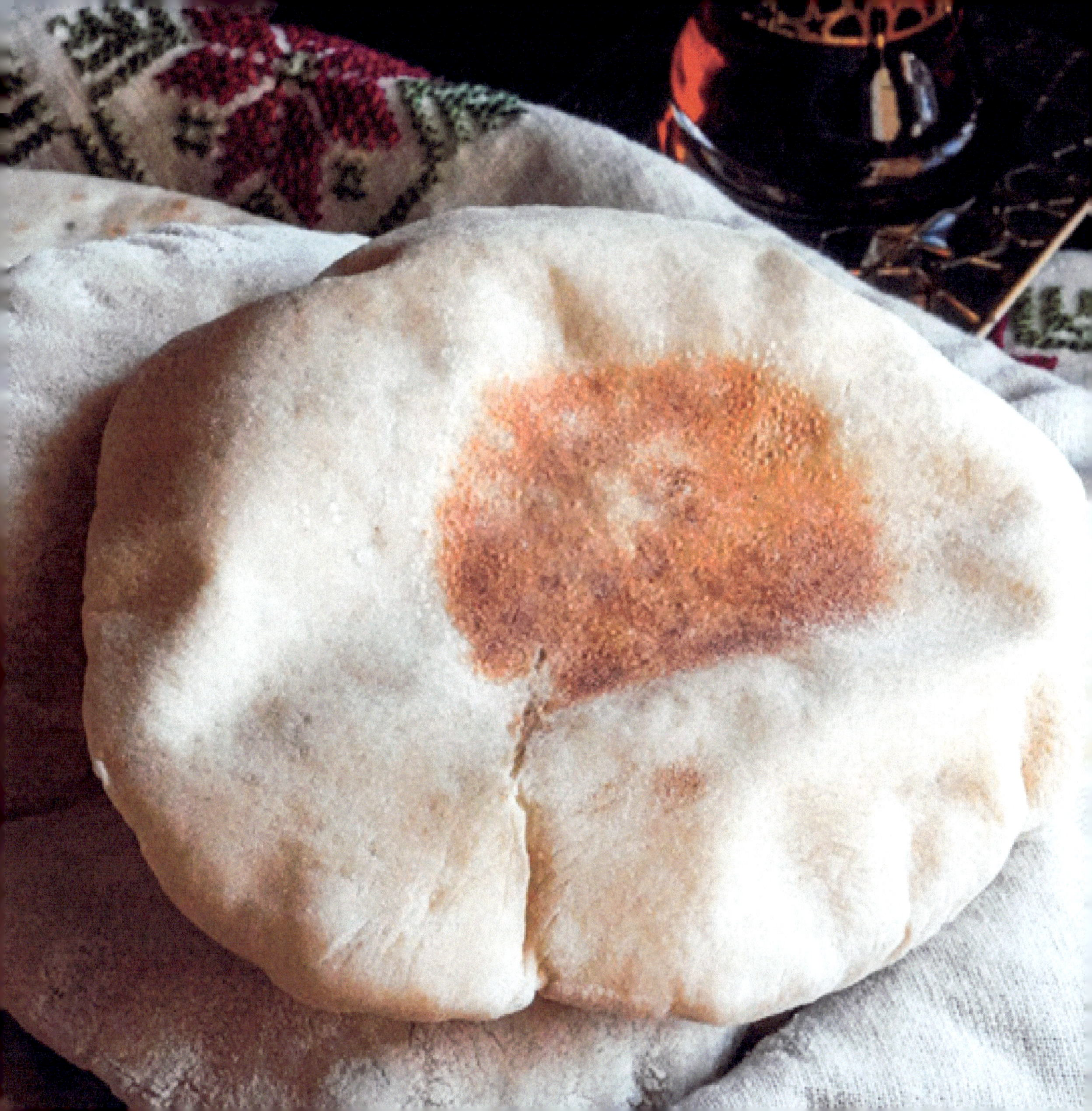

Za'atar زعتر

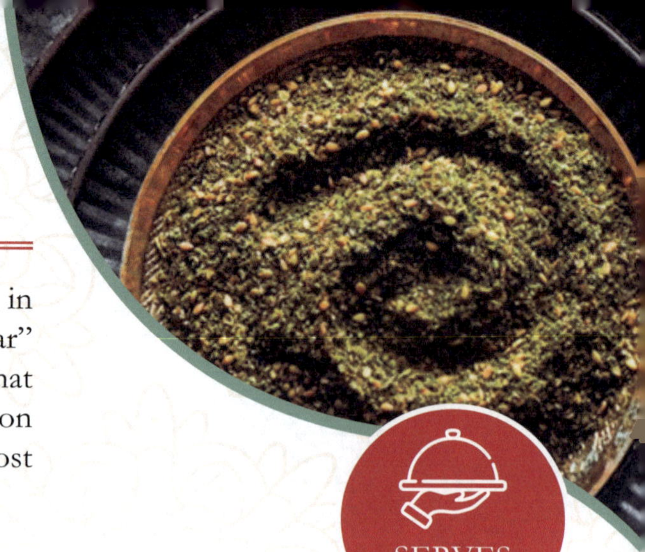

Za'atar is a versatile and aromatic spice blend that is widely used in Middle Eastern cuisine, originating in Palestine. The term "zaatar" can refer to both the spice blend itself and to a specific herb that is part of the mixture. The blend typically includes a combination of dried herbs, spices, and sometimes seeds. This is how most Palestinians make it, and you can customize it to your liking.

SERVES

INGREDIENTS:

- 2 cups zaatar leaves (thyme, zaatar herb)
- 3 tbsp sumac
- 4 tbsp toasted sesame seeds
- ¾ tsp salt, or to taste
- 1 tbsp extra virgin olive oil

DIRECTIONS:

It's important to use a spice grinder rather than a food processor in this case.

1. Toast the sesame seeds in a pan on medium heat until golden in color. Set aside to cool.
2. Add the zaatar leaves in batches into your spice grinder. Grind until slightly coarse but mostly fine. If you like it more on the powdery side, grind it until completely fine. Repeat until all the za'atar is finished.
3. Add the toasted sesame seeds and ground zaatar to a bowl. Add the salt and sumac, and mix. You can adjust the saltiness here.
4. Add the tbsp of olive oil and rub it well using your hands.
5. Mix well and store in an airtight container.

Pro Tip: Using good quality sumac means not needing to add lemon juice. Authentic zaatar only has these ingredients, plus possibly adding cumin for taste.

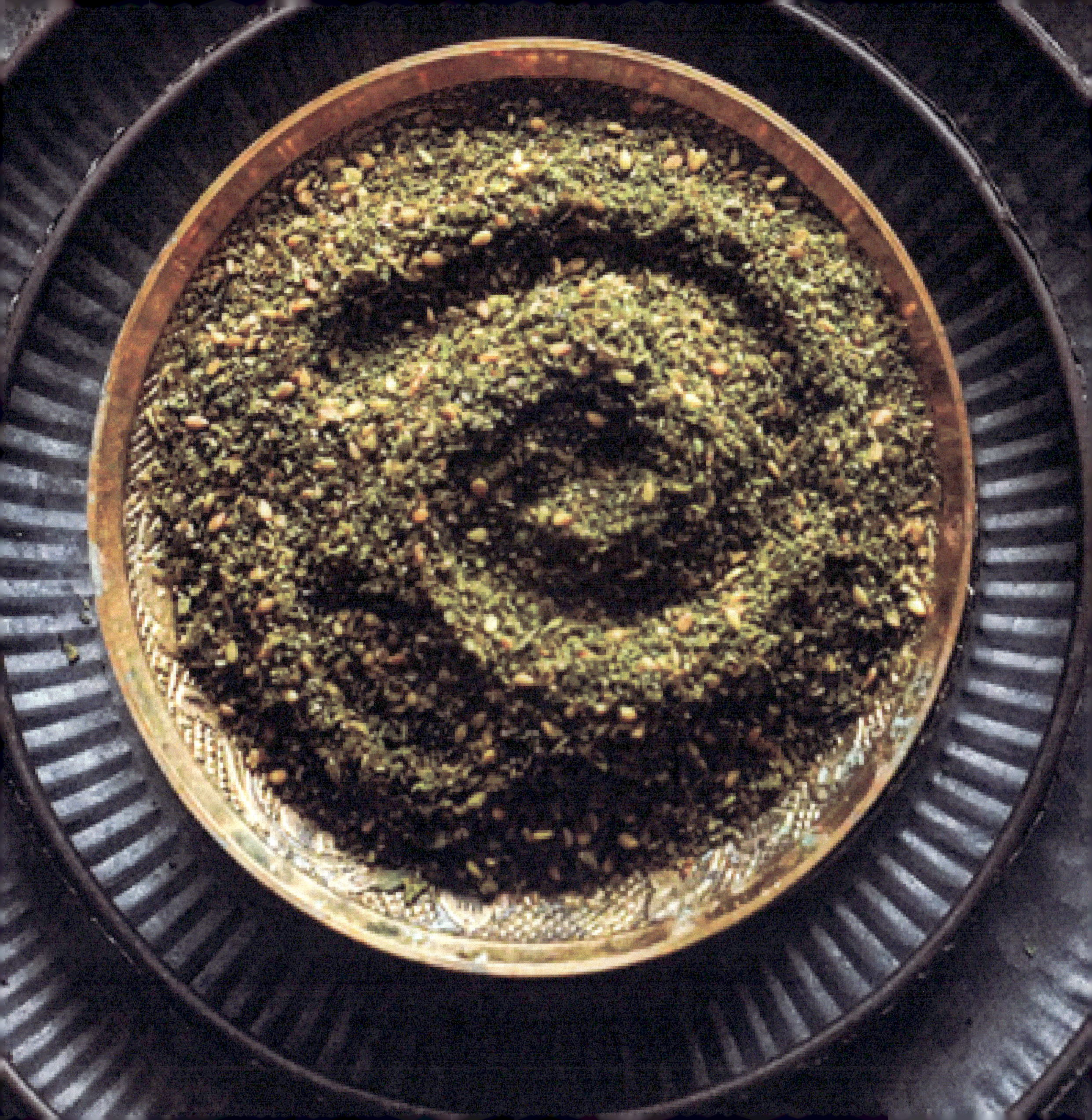

Qishta Arabiya قشطة عربية

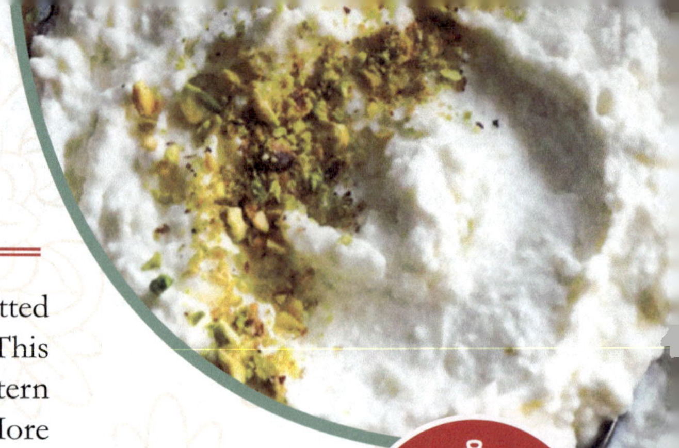

SERVES

Qishta, also known as Ashta, is a traditional Middle Eastern clotted cream that holds a special place in the region's culinary heritage. This rich and creamy dairy product is a staple in many Middle Eastern desserts, providing a luscious texture and a distinctive flavor. More often than not, it is made the quicker way without using cheese curds, but this is the more rich and flavorful version. This can be used for any and all desserts calling for qishta, or eat it on its own with honey.

INGREDIENTS:

Cheese:

- 4 cups whole milk
- ¼ cup white vinegar

Cream:

- 1¼ cups heavy cream
- ¾ cup whole milk
- ¼ cup granulated sugar
- 2½ tbsp cornstarch
- ½ tsp orange blossom water
- 2 crushed mastic rocks

DIRECTIONS:

1. Add the milk to a pot on low heat, let it simmer gently.
2. Once it starts to slightly bubble around the edges, add the vinegar. Stir until it begins clotting. Keep stirring to encourage clotting.
3. Remove the curds using a slotted spoon and transfer to a bowl. Cover until cooled.
4. Prepare the cream. In a saucepan, without turning on the heat, combine the heavy whipping cream, whole milk, and cornstarch. Whisk together well until the cornstarch is dissolved and no longer clumpy.
5. Put the mastic with a small pinch of sugar and crush using a mortar and pestle. Make sure no large chunks remain and it's completely ground.
6. Add the sauce pan to the stove on medium-high heat. Add the granulated sugar and the crushed mastic and whisk. Continuously whisk until the mixture thickens, about 10 minutes. You want to continuously whisk so the bottom doesn't burn.

7. Once thick, add in the orange blossom and give it one final stir.
8. Transfer the qishta to a flat plate and cover with plastic wrap so it doesn't develop a crust. Refrigerate until completely cooled.
9. Once the cream and the cheese are both cooled, mix together to combine. You could add both to a food processor to make the mixture more smooth, but it will make it a little less stiff to work with.

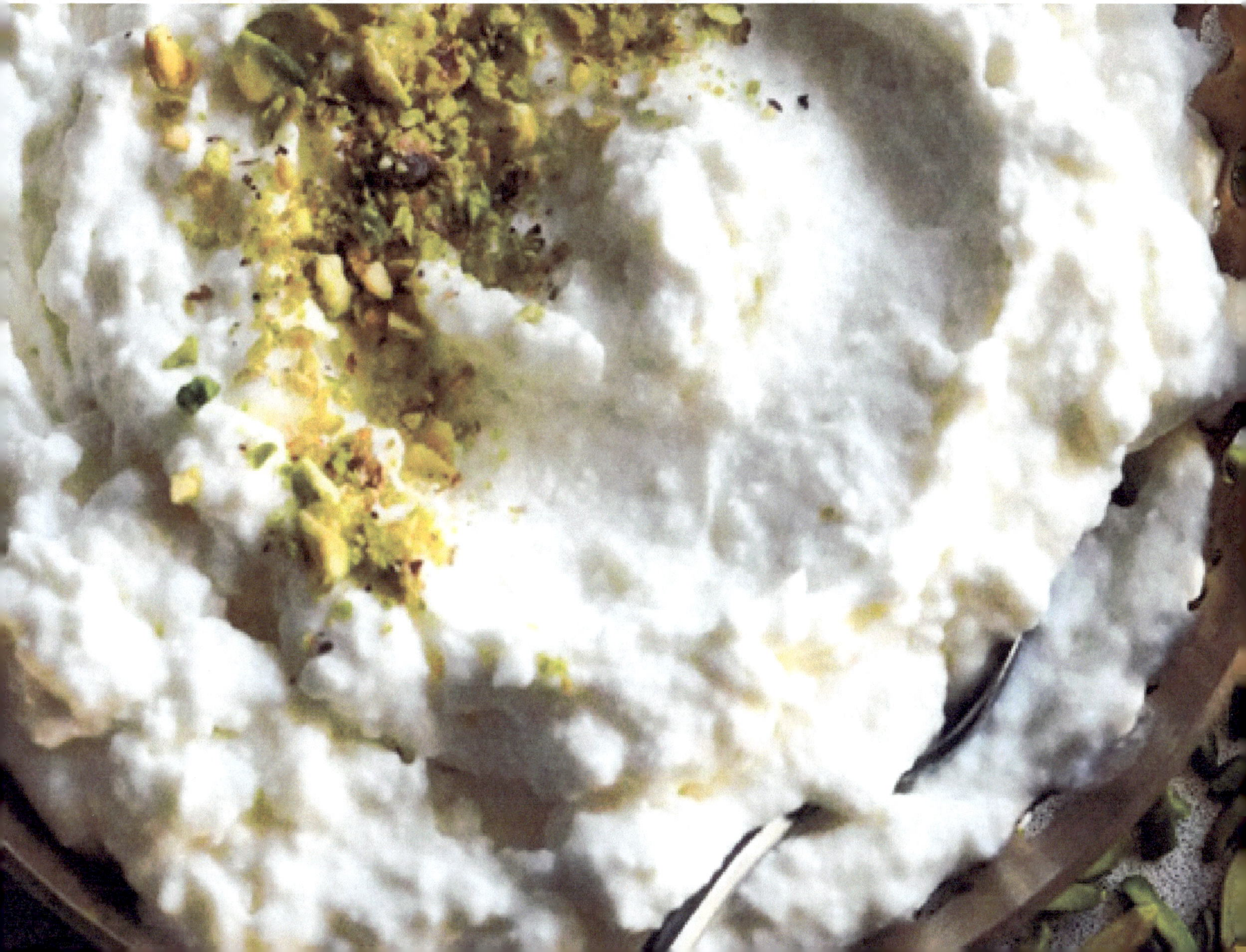

Arab Desserts And Treats

حلويات ومشروبات عربية

Arab desserts invite you to experience the magic of flavors that transcend boundaries, telling a story of cultural richness and the deep-rooted connection between sweetness and hospitality. Join us on this delectable exploration, where every dessert is a celebration of tradition and the sweet legacy passed down through generations.

From street carts selling Sahlab and Balah El Sham to dessert shops piling on the Baklawa sky high. Arab desserts are the greatest in the world, and they're right at your fingertips

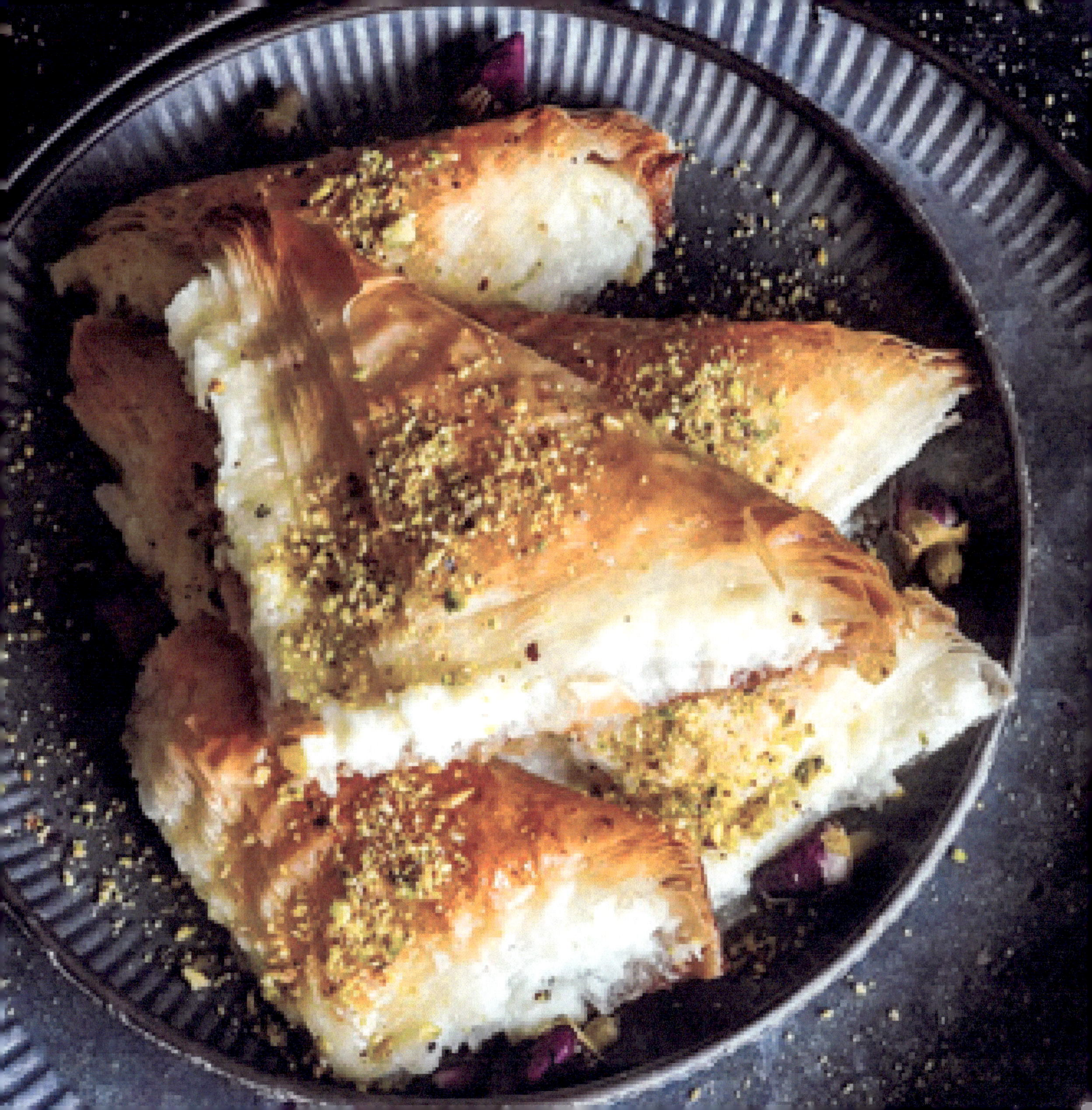

Rose and Cardamom Muhallabia مهلبية

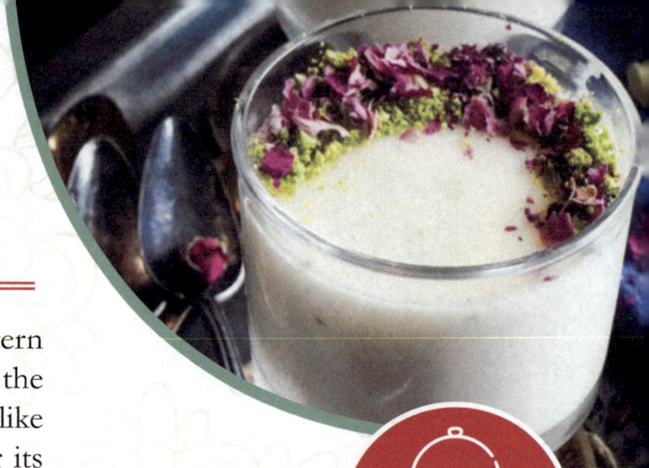

SERVES
4

Rose and Cardamom Muhallabieh is a delightful Middle Eastern dessert that combines the fragrant essence of rose water with the warm, citrusy notes of cardamom. This traditional pudding-like dish, also known as Mahalabia or Muhallebi, is appreciated for its smooth and creamy texture, and its easy preparation.

INGREDIENTS:

- 4 cups cold heavy whipping cream
- ¼ cup cornstarch
- ½ -⅔ cup granulated sugar (depending on desired sweetness)
- ¼ tsp crushed mastic rocks
- 1 tsp freshly ground cardamom
- 1 tsp rose water

DIRECTIONS:

1. Without turning on the stove, combine the cornstarch and cold heavy cream in a pot. Whisk together well, ensuring no clumps of cornstarch remain.
2. Add the pot to the stove on medium-high heat.
3. Putthe mastic rocks with a pinch of sugar and crush using a mortar and pestle. Make sure they're finely crushed and without any large pieces.
4. Add the crushed mastic, along with the ½ cup sugar and ground cardamom to the pot.
5. Continuously whisk to ensure the bottom doesn't burn or clump. This needs a little patience. It should start thickening after about 8-12 minutes.
6. Stir in the rose water. Immediately divide into 4 serving bowls and refrigerate until cold.
7. Garnish with edible rose petals and ground pistachios.

Pro Tips:

» If you like a lighter rose flavor, add it when whisking in the sugar and mastic.

» If you do not like rose and cardamom flavors, you could use orange blossom water, or even vanilla extract.

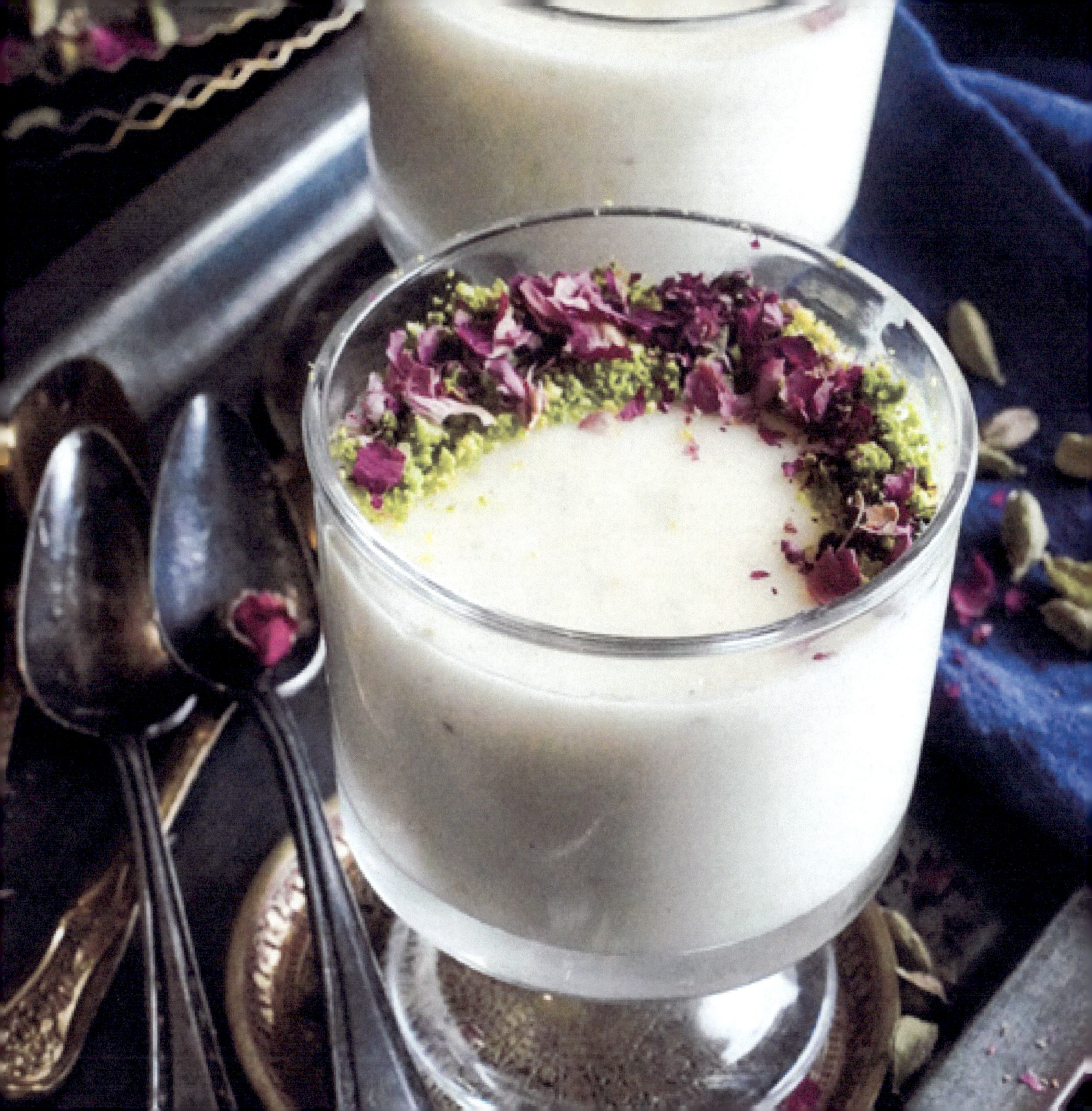

Baklawa Cheesecake Bars

تشيز كيك البقلاوة

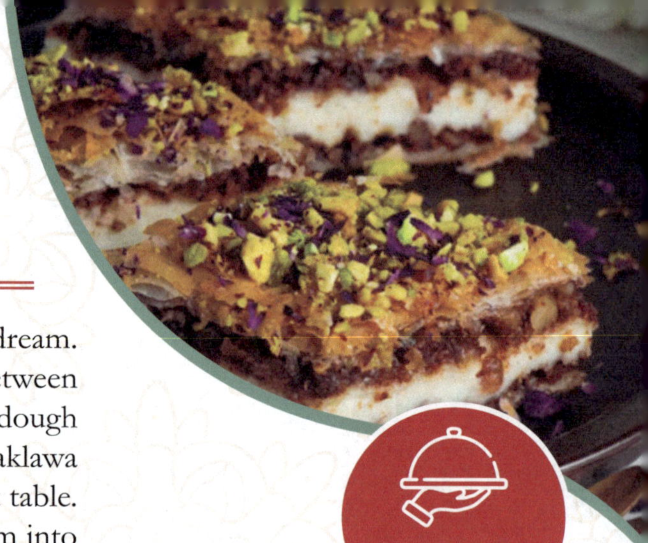

SERVES

These utterly delicious Baklava Cheesecake Bars are an absolute dream. The combination of decadent and creamy cheesecake nestled between two layers of cinnamon walnut baklava and crispy, buttery phyllo dough is something you'll never get tired of. These show-stopping baklawa cheesecake minis will steal the show at every dinner and dessert table. They're also the perfect size to feed a crowd, as you can cut them into desired size.

INGREDIENTS:

Cheesecake Batter:

- 16 oz cream cheese, room temperature (450g)
- 3 tbsp sour cream, room temperature
- 3 tbsp milk or heavy cream
- 1½ tbsp all purpose flour
- 2 large eggs, room temperature (140g)
- 1 tsp rosewater
- ⅔ cup granulated sugar

Baklava Filling:

- 3 cups chopped walnuts
- ¾ cup granulated sugar
- 1 tsp orange blossom water
- 1 tsp rose water
- 1½ tablespoons ground cinnamon

Phyllo Layers:

- 1 lb Phyllo dough, about 28-32 sheets
- 1½ sticks unsalted butter melted
- Simple syrup for serving

DIRECTIONS:

Prepare the simple syrup ahead of time so it has time to cool.

1. Preheat the oven to 350°F.
2. Make sure the cream cheese, eggs, and sour cream are at room temperature, and that the phyllo is thawed according to package instructions.

3. To a bowl of a stand mixer and using a paddle attachment, add the cream cheese and sugar and beat on medium speed until smooth, about 3-5 minutes. Stop and scrape down the sides.
4. Return to medium speed and add the sour cream, rosewater, cream or milk, and flour. Beat until smooth. Scrape down the sides and return to medium-low speed.
5. Add the eggs, and beat just until incorporated. Do not over mix or your cheesecake will be gritty and gummy.

Baklava Filling:

1. Add the walnuts to a food processor or chop by hand until slightly chunky but not fine.
2. Transfer to a bowl and add the cinnamon, rose water, orange blossom and sugar. Mix and set aside.

Assembly:

1. Take a 9×13 pan and brush it with 2 tablespoons of melted butter. Add 1 sheet of phyllo dough and brush with butter. Repeat phyllo layers until you reach 8.
2. Now, add 1 cup of the walnut baklava filling, make sure to spread it evenly. Top with 5 sheets of phyllo dough, brushing with butter in between each layer.
3. Now, add the cheesecake batter on top, spreading it around evenly.
4. Add 1 sheet of phyllo dough on top and brush with melted butter. Repeat until 5 sheets are finished.
5. Add the remaining walnut baklava filling on top.
6. Top with the remaining phyllo dough sheets, brushing with butter in between each layer.
7. Bake at 350° for about 40-50 minutes, or until golden.
8. Remove from the oven and immediately top with simple syrup, about 2 cups.
9. Let it cool at room temp for 1 hour before refrigerating 6 hours uncovered, preferably overnight.
10. Slice carefully with a sharp knife and serve with more syrup and chopped pistachios, and enjoy.

Pro Tips:

- Count your phyllo dough sheet and divide them in half. My package had 28. I used 14 for the bottom layer and 14 for the top.
- It's essential to let it cool for a long time in the fridge to ensure even and smooth cuts, and to make sure the cheesecake filling sets.

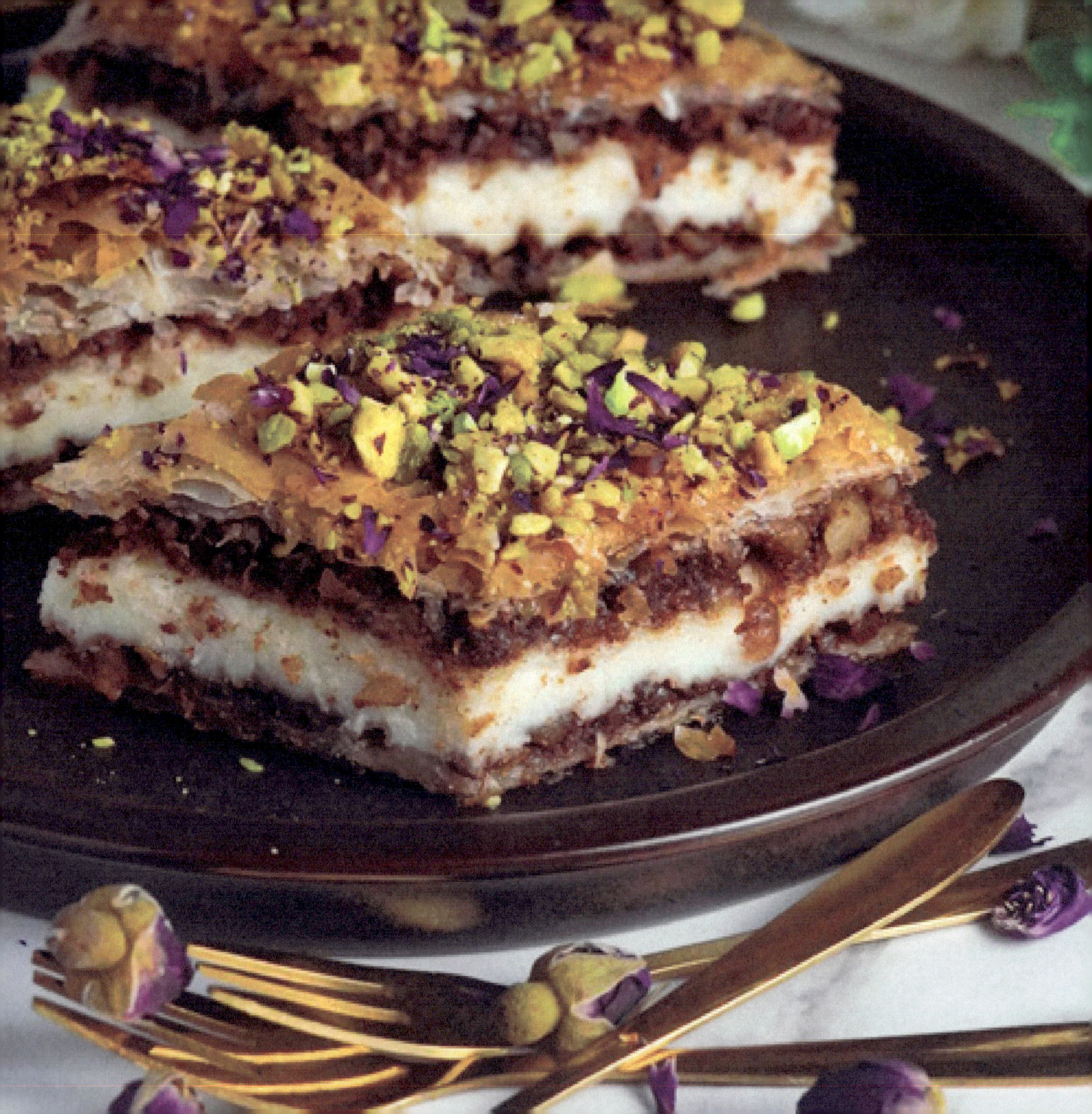

Balah El Sham (Tulumba)

بلح الشام

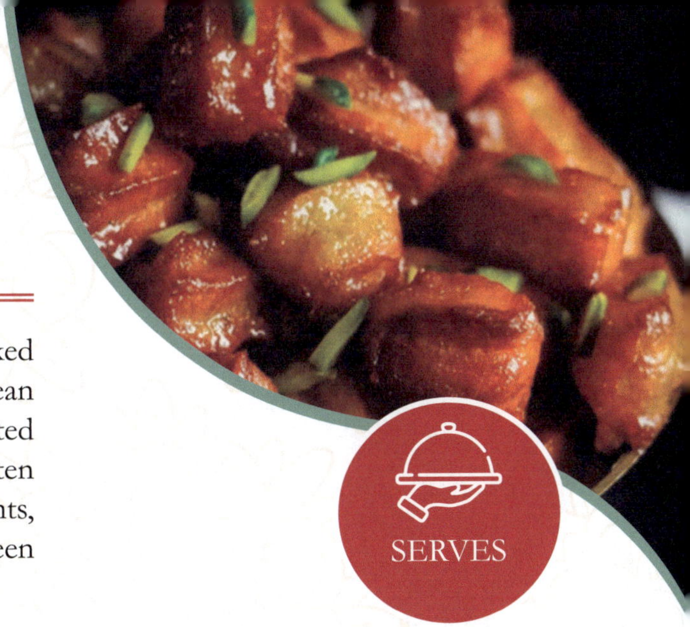

SERVES

Balah El Sham, or Tulumba, is a popular sweet and syrup-soaked dessert that is enjoyed in various Middle Eastern and Mediterranean countries. This deep-fried pastry is characterized by its elongated and cylindrical shape, resembling small tubes or fingers. It is often found at festive occasions, celebrations, and during special events, and often sold on street carts. They're the perfect cross between crunchy and soft, and they're absolutely delicious.

INGREDIENTS:

- 2 cups all purpose flour
- 2 tbsp cornstarch
- ¼ tsp salt
- 1½ tbsp sugar
- 3 large eggs
- 1 cup whole milk
- ¼ cup water
- ⅓ cup neutral oil, such as avocado or canola oil
- More oil, for frying

Qater (simple syrup):

- 3 cups granulated sugar
- 2 cups water
- 1 tbsp lemon juice
- 1 tsp orange blossom water

DIRECTIONS:

1. Prepare the simple syrup. Start by combining the granulated sugar and water in a pot, and place them on high heat. Let the mixture come to a boil.
2. Once boiled for 10 minutes, add in the lemon juice and the orange blossom water.
3. Stir, and set aside to cool completely at room temperature.
4. Begin by adding the milk, water, and oil to a saucepan on medium heat.
5. Let it heat up for a few minutes until it starts to bubble.
6. In the meantime, combine together the all purpose flour, cornstarch, sugar, and salt. Mix them well.

7. Once the liquids are bubbling, stir in the dry ingredients and mix well. Once well-mixed, remove from the stove and let it cool down completely.
8. Once the mixture is completely cooled, add in the eggs. You can use an electric whisk to make it easier.
9. Heat up enough oil on medium heat to deep fry the pastries, about 6. It should reach 350 F.
10. Transfer the pastry mixture to a piping bag fitted with a star piping tip.
11. Once the oil is hot, grab the piping bag and a pair of kitchen shears. Pipe a straight line into the oil, about 1½ to 2 inches in length, and use the shears to cut it off from the piping tip end. Repeat until the frying pan is full.
12. Fry until golden brown, then immediately dip into the simple syrup for a minute before transferring them to a plate.

Serve garnished with ground pistachios. These are best eaten immediately.

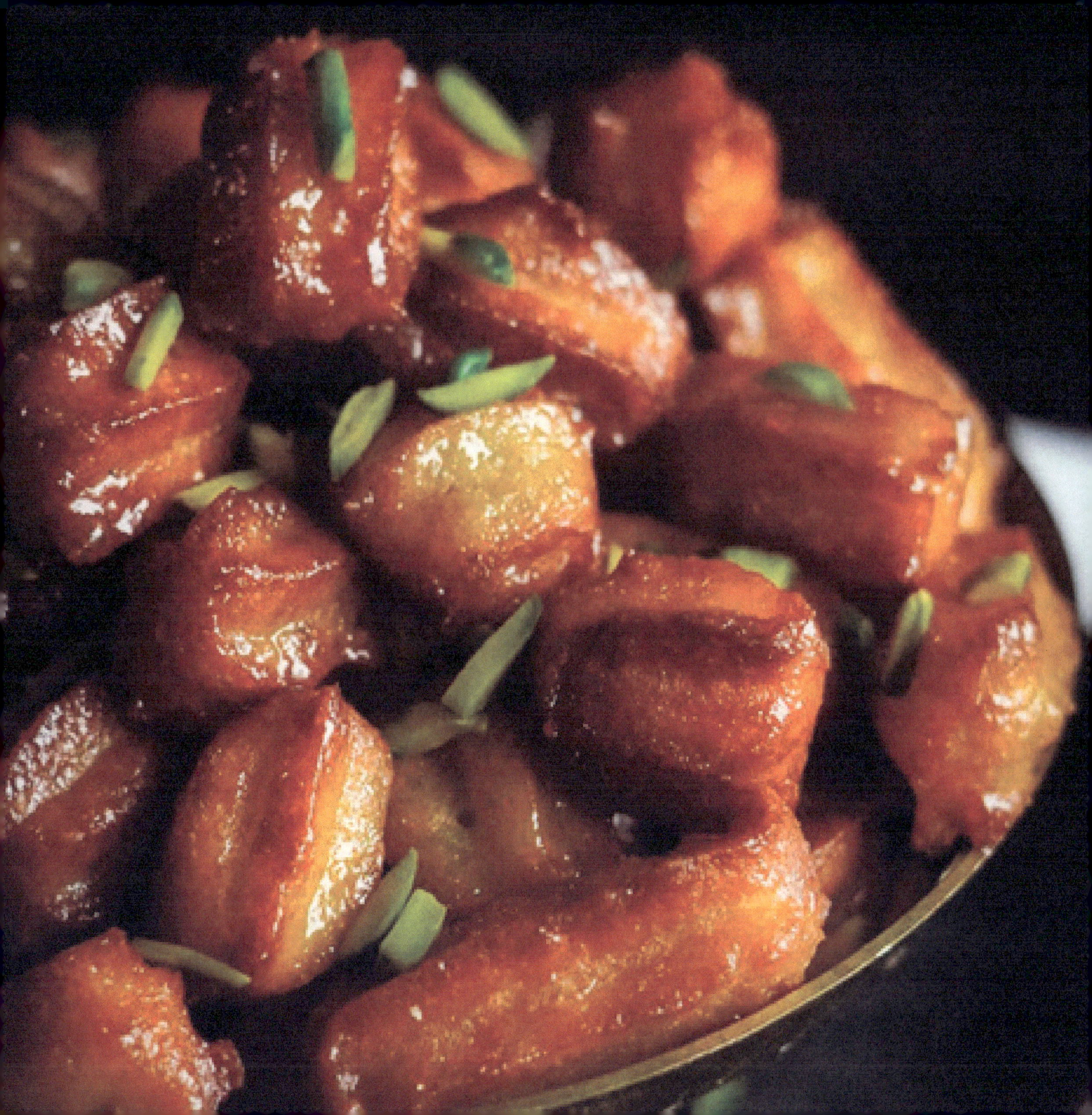

Pistachio Mafroukeh مفروكة بالفستق

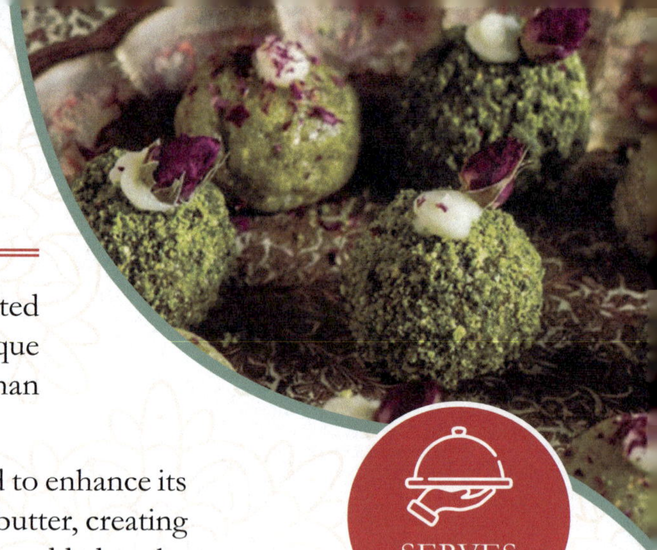

Mafroukeh is a traditional Middle Eastern dessert that originated in Lebanon. This sweet and nutty treat is known for its unique combination of semolina, sugar, and various nuts, more often than not, pistachios.

The main component of mafroukeh is semolina, which is roasted to enhance its nutty flavor. This roasted semolina is then mixed with sugar and butter, creating a crumbly and slightly sandy texture. Finely ground pistachios are added to the mixture, providing a delightful crunch and additional depth of flavor.

SERVES

INGREDIENTS:

- Pistachio Shell:
- 2 tbsp unsalted butter
- 3 cups coarse semolina
- 1 cup water
- 1 ¼ cup granulated sugar
- 1 tbsp orange blossom water
- 1 ½ cups finely ground pistachios

Qishta:

- 2 cups heavy whipping cream
- ⅔ cups granulated sugar
- 4 tbsp cornstarch
- 1½ tsp orange blossom water

DIRECTIONS:

1. Prepare the qishta. In a saucepan, without turning on the heat, combine the heavy whipping cream and cornstarch. Whisk together well until the cornstarch is dissolved and no longer clumpy.
2. Add the sauce pan to the stove on medium-high heat. Add the granulated sugar and whisk. Continuously whisk until the mixture thickens, about 10 minutes. You want to continuously whisk so the bottom doesn't burn.
3. Once thick, add in the orange blossom and give it one final stir.

4. Transfer the qishta to a flat plate and cover with plastic wrap so it doesn't develop a crust. Refrigerate until completely cooled.
5. In another pot on medium heat, melt the unsalted butter. Add the semolina and toast until it's toasted but not burnt, about 3-5 minutes. Set aside.
6. In another saucepan, combine the water and sugar and let it come to a boil. Once bubbling, immediately stir in the toasted semolina and the ground pistachios. Fold until well combined.
7. Let it cool at room temperature, covered.
8. Once cooled, grab a small ping pong sized ball of dough. Poke your thumb in the center to make a well. Grab a small ball of cooled qishta and add it to the center, and seal the ball back up.
9. Dip the sealed ball into finely ground pistachios and serve.

If you have a sweet tooth, you can also serve with some simple syrup.

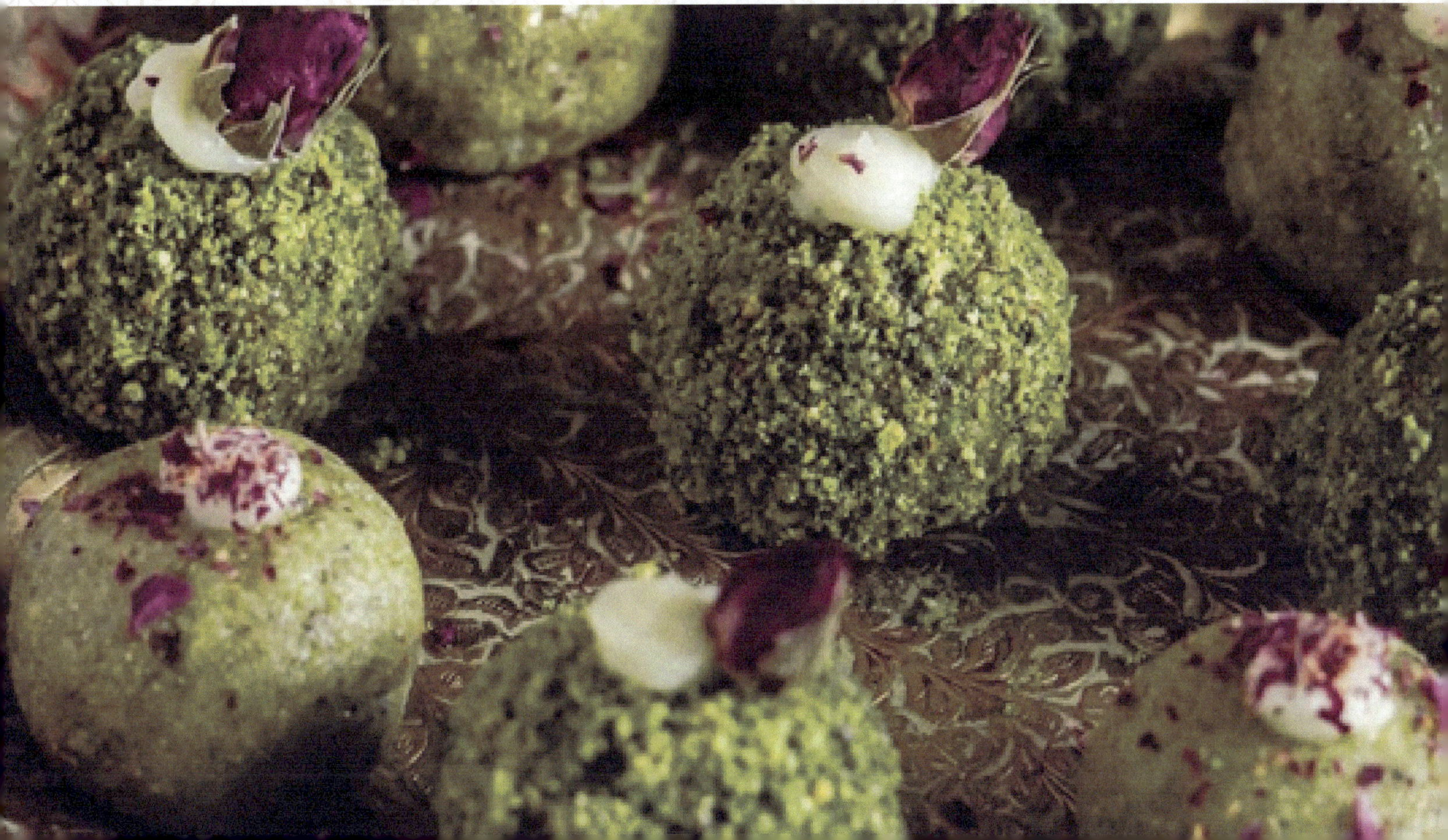

Qatayef قطايف

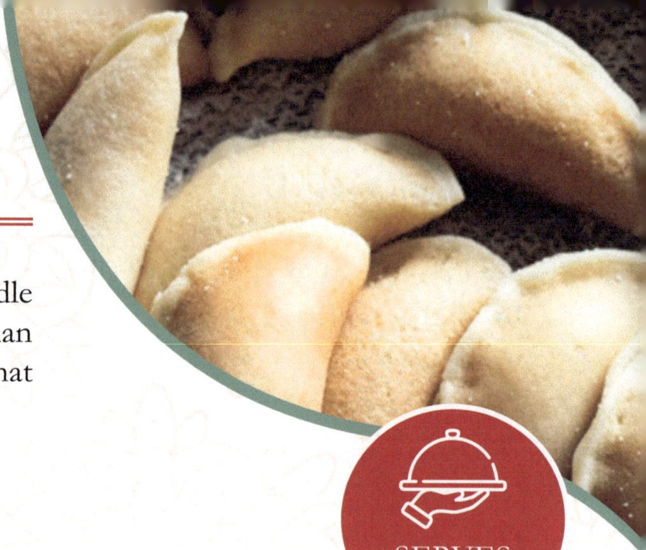

Qatayef, also known as Katayef or Atayef, is a popular Middle Eastern dessert, commonly enjoyed during the month of Ramadan and other festive occasions. It is a type of pancake or dumpling that can be filled with cheese, nuts, or qishta.

SERVES

INGREDIENTS:

- 1 ½ cups all purpose flour
- 1 cup fine semolina
- 1 tbsp baking powder
- ½ tsp yeast
- 3 tbsp sugar
- ⅛ tsp salt
- 1 tsp orange blossom water, optional
- 3 cups lukewarm water

Cheese Filling:

- Ackawi or panela, or sweet cheese.

To Serve:

- Simple syrup for serving
- Pistachios

DIRECTIONS:

1. Sift the flour, sugar, baking powder, semolina, yeast, and salt into a blender.
2. Add the lukewarm water. If you're using orange blossom or rose water, add it now too.
3. Blend for 2 minutes, then let it sit for half an hour covered.
4. Once rested, blend again for 30 seconds to deflate the batter.
5. Preheat your skillet or griddle on medium- high heat. It should be hot.
6. Pour the qatayef into the desired size.
7. Wait for the surface to dry. It should have holes all over the top, do not flip it. You want the surface to look more matte than shiny and wet. Remove the qatayef piece using a flat spatula and place onto a clean towel. Do not flip.
8. Cover them with a towel so as to not dry out until ready for filling.
9. For the cheese filling, I use whole milk panela, or ackawi, or Chicago cheese.

10. Stuff the qatayef with the shredded or broken apart cheese making sure to not overstuff.
11. Do not forget to seal well by pinching the edges shut.
12. Fry in oil preheated on medium heat until golden. Alternatively, you can bake them after brushing them in oil on both sides until crispy, for about 20 minutes at 450F, flipping halfway, then immediately dunk them in simple syrup.

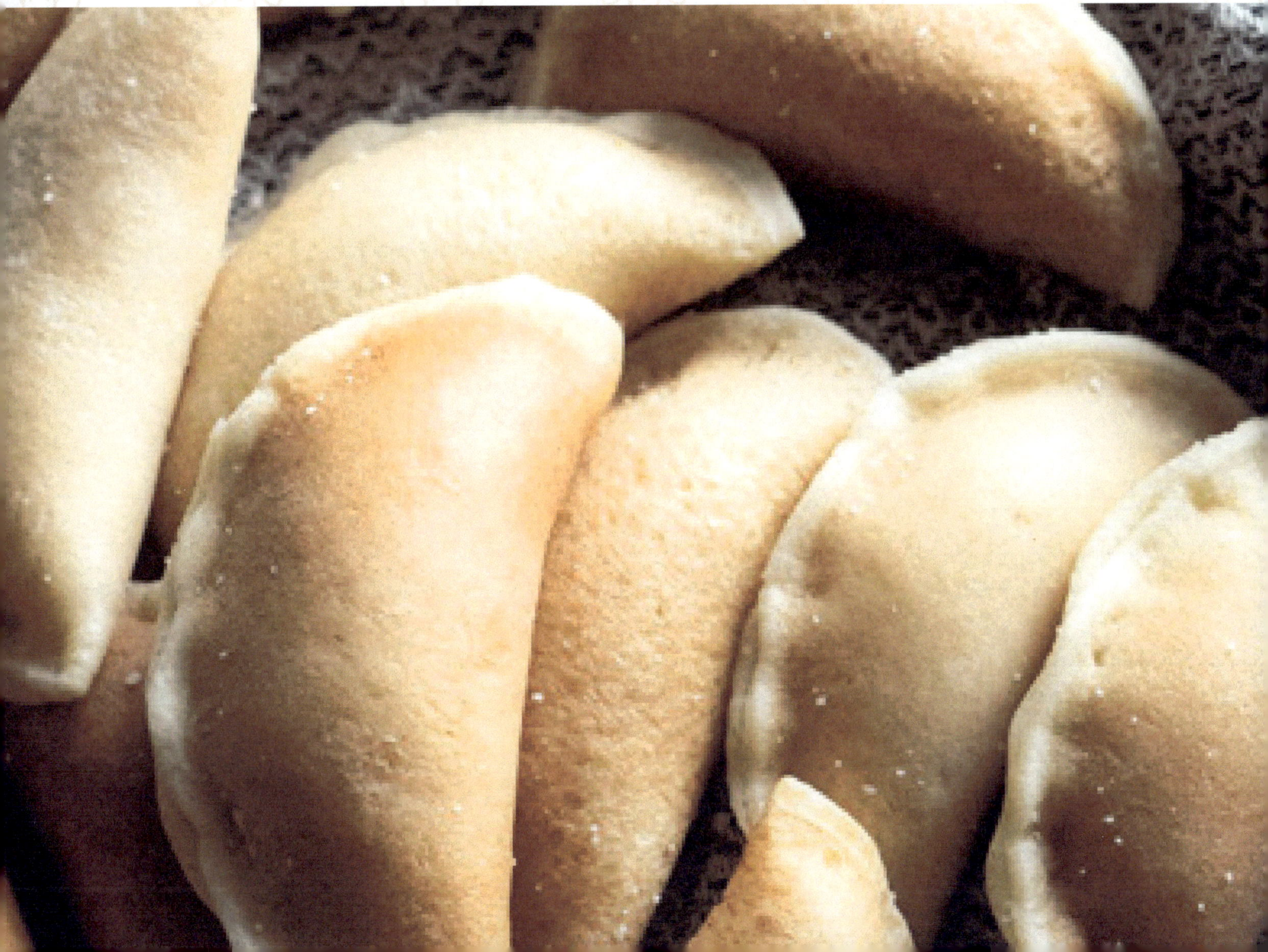

Sfouf صفوف

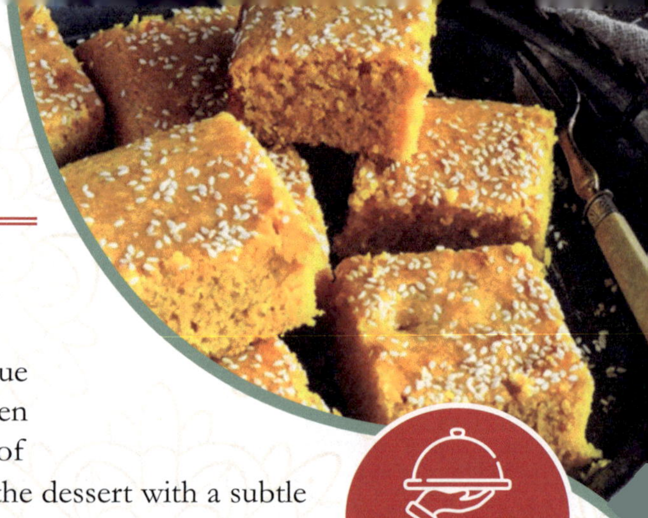

(Lebanese Turmeric Cake)

Sfouf is a delightful Lebanese dessert that stands out for its unique combination of flavors and textures. This yellow-hued cake, often referred to as "Turmeric Cake," is characterized by the inclusion of turmeric, which not only lends a vibrant color but also infuses the dessert with a subtle earthy flavor. This moist and spongy cake is sweetened with a generous amount of sugar and enriched with semolina. It's moist, delicious, and so addicting.

SERVES
9 Pieces

INGREDIENTS:

- 1 cup All Purpose flour, spooned and leveled
- 1 cup fine semolina
- ¾ tsp baking powder
- 1 tbsp turmeric
- 1 cup granulated sugar
- ¼ tsp salt
- 1 tsp vanilla extract
- ½ cup plain whole milk yogurt
- ½ cup whole milk
- ½ cup neutral oil, like avocado or canola
- 1 ½ tbsp tahini paste
- Sesame seeds or pine nuts, for topping

DIRECTIONS:

1. Preheat oven to 350 F
2. In a bowl, combine the 1 cup all purpose flour, 1 cup fine semolina, and ¾ teaspoon baking powder. Mix in the ¼ teaspoon salt and 1 tablespoon turmeric.
3. In another bowl, combine together the 1 cup sugar, the ½ cup milk, ½ cup plain yogurt, and the ½ cup oil. Drizzle in the vanilla extract and whisk together well, until well combined.
4. Add the dry ingredients into the wet mixture and whisk well.
5. Prepare a 9x9 inch pan and brush with the 1 ½ tablespoons of tahini paste, making sure to get it all around the pan.
6. Add the batter and smooth the top.

7. Sprinkle the top with sesame seeds, or pine nuts, or leave as is.
8. Bake at 350 F for 25-35 minutes, or until a toothpick comes out clean. I prefer to broil it for 2 minutes or so to brown it.
9. Allow it to completely cool at room temperature before cutting and serving.

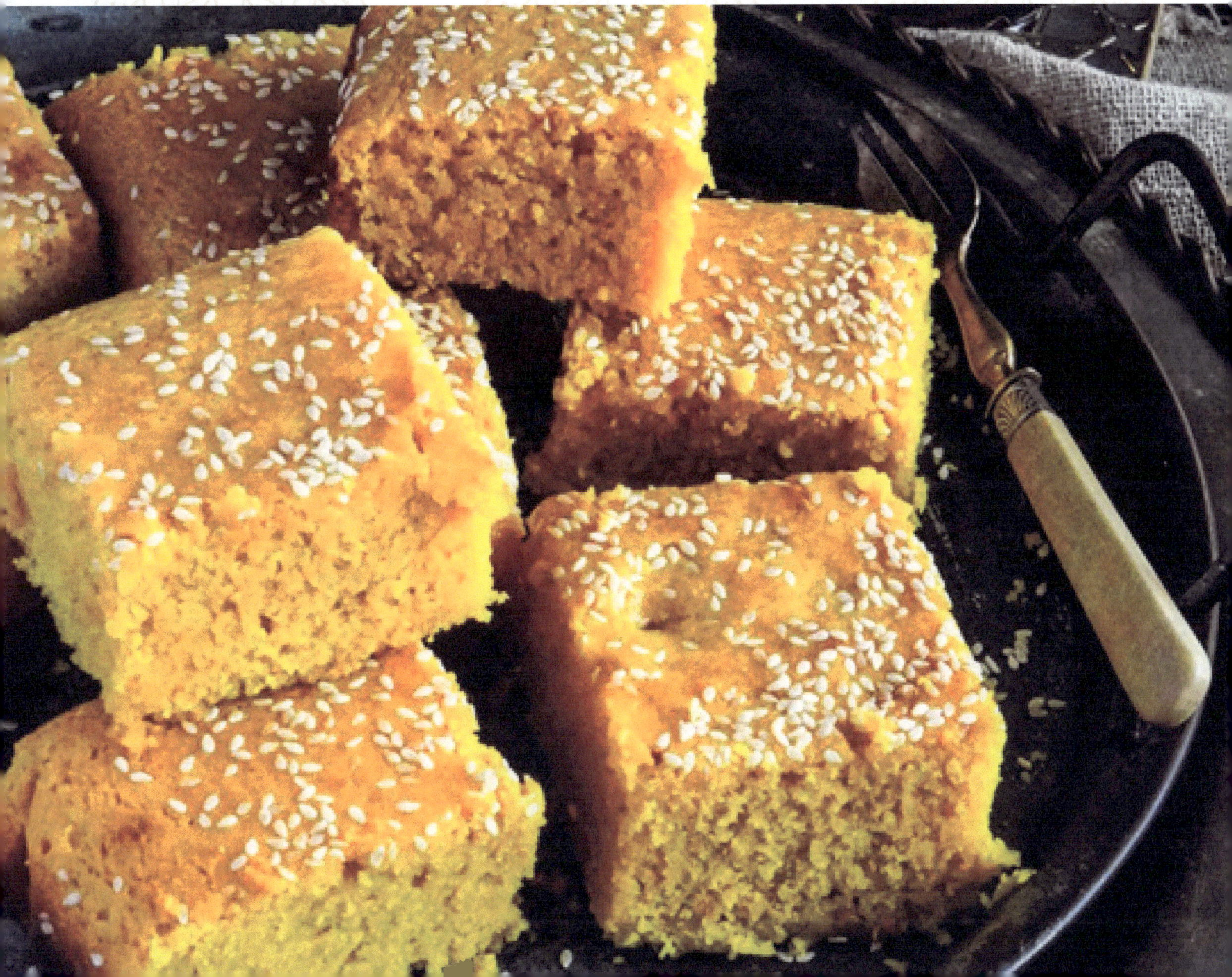

Simsimyeh سمسمية

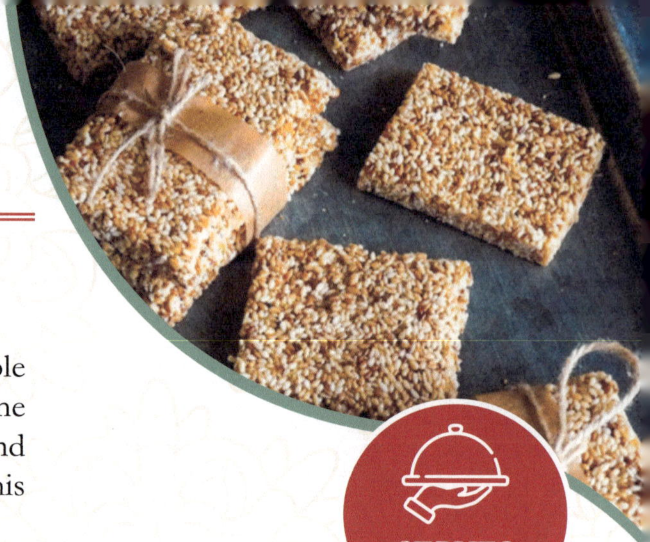

SERVES

(Sesame Candy)

Middle Eastern sesame candy, Simsimyeh,is a delightful and simple sweet treat that showcases the rich and nutty flavor of sesame seeds. This candy is widely enjoyed across the Middle East and is known for its crunchy texture and sweet taste. Oftentimes, this dessert is made and distributed during cultural celebrations.

INGREDIENTS:

- ½ cup granulated sugar
- ½ cup honey
- 2½ cups toasted sesame seeds

DIRECTIONS:

1. To begin, start by adding the sesame seeds to a pan on high heat. Once you see some color develop, lower the heat to low and continuously stir until the sesame seeds are a toasted brown color. Set aside.
2. Lay flat 2 rectangular pieces of parchment paper. Lightly brush or spray with oil. Grease a sharp knife and set aside.
3. Add the sugar and honey to a saucepan on medium heat. Mix well.
4. Once the honey and sugar mixture looks bubbly, immediately remove and pour on top of the toasted sesame seeds.
5. Mix everything together well using a rubber spatula until everything is well combined.
6. Pour the sesame mixture on top of one greased parchment paper.
7. Place the other greased parchment paper right on top of the sesame mixture and roll it thinner using a rolling pin.
8. Remove the top piece of parchment paper, and cut the sesame candy using the greased knife. Trim the edges for cleaner cuts and pieces.
9. Let it completely cool before cutting once again to get nice looking pieces.

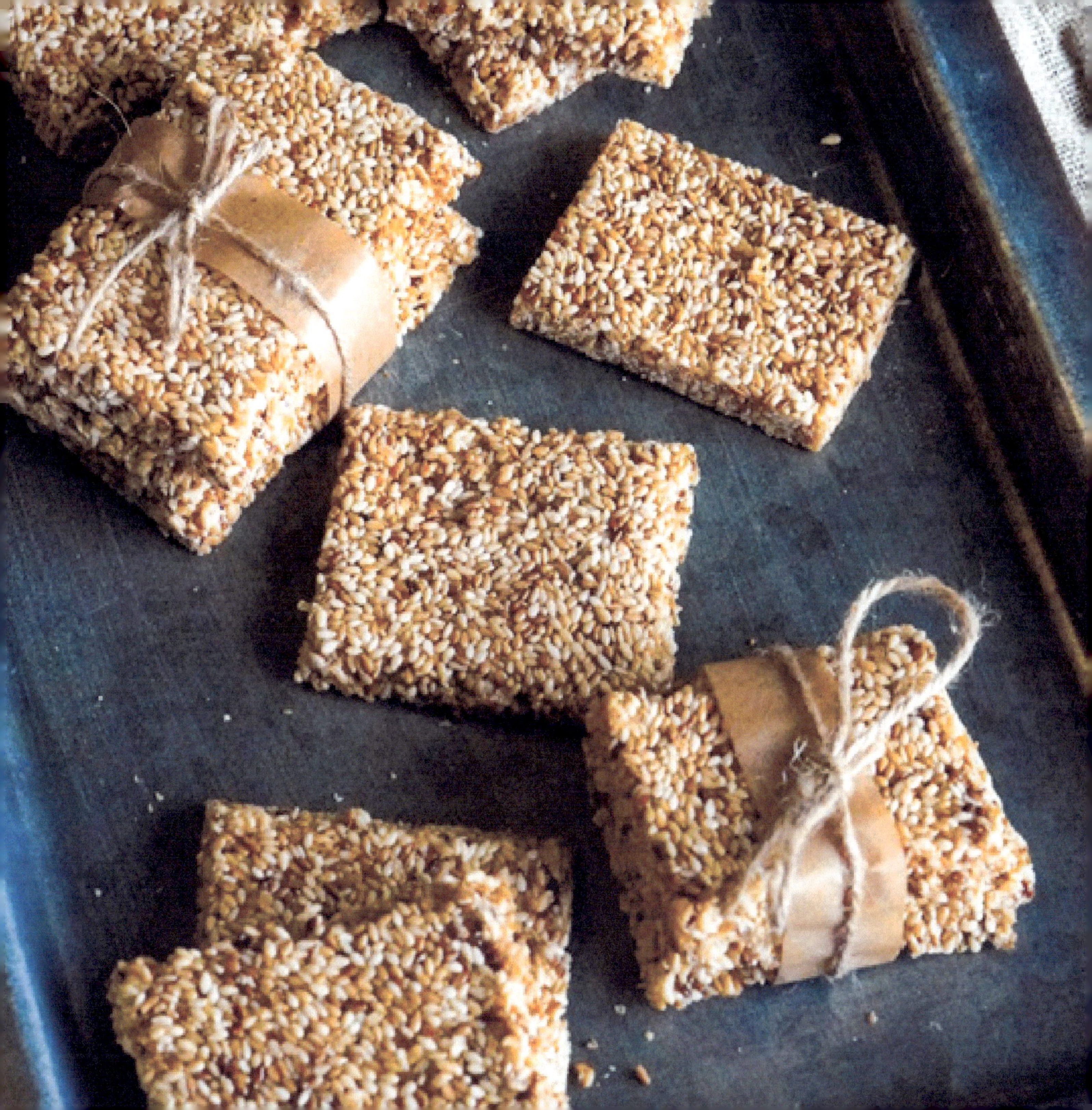

Um Ali أم علي

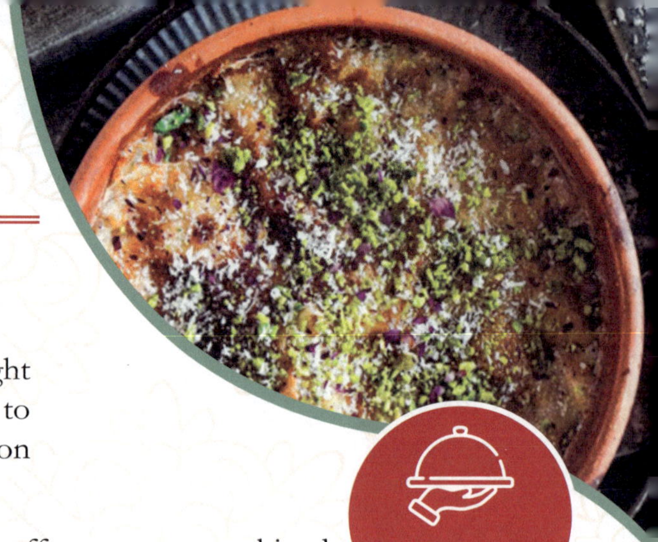

(Egyptian Bread Pudding)

Um Ali, a classic Egyptian dessert, is a rich and indulgent delight that weaves together layers of flavor and texture. Often referred to as "Mother of Ali," this dessert has a history steeped in tradition and is a staple in Egyptian households.

At its core, Um Ali is a bread pudding, where layers of flaky puff pastry are combined with a luscious mixture of cream and sugar. The dessert is generously spiced with aromatic additions such as cinnamon and cardamom, infusing each layer with warmth and sweetness.

SERVES 4-6

INGREDIENTS:

- 1 package puff pastry (490g)
- 5 cups heavy whipping cream
- 1 ¼ cups granulated sugar
- ½ tsp ground cardamom
- ½ tsp ground cinnamon
- 1 cinnamon stick

Topping:

- 1 cup heavy cream
- 1 tbsp granulated sugar
- 1 tsp vanilla extract

Garnish:

- Ground pistachios
- Coconut flakes

DIRECTIONS:

1. Preheat oven to 400 F
2. Thaw the puff pastry according to package instructions, but keep cold. Cut the puff pastry into squares. Place flat into a lined baking sheet, and bake at 400 F for 15-25 minutes, or until golden. Remove and set aside.
3. In a saucepan on the stove, combine the 5 cups of heavy whipping cream along with the granulated sugar, cinnamon stick, ground cinnamon and ground cardamom. Stir on medium heat until the sugar is dissolved and the cream is well heated, almost boiling.

4. Break apart about ¾ of the baked puff pastry into a 9x13 pan.
5. Pour the spiced hot heavy cream mixture on top. Add pistachios and shredded coconuts, as desired.
6. Top with the remaining amount of broken puff pastry on top. Smash it down lightly with a spoon.
7. Return the Um Ali tray into the oven, and broil on the middle rack at 400 F until the pan begins to bubble.
8. Remove from the oven, and garnish with more pistachios or nuts.

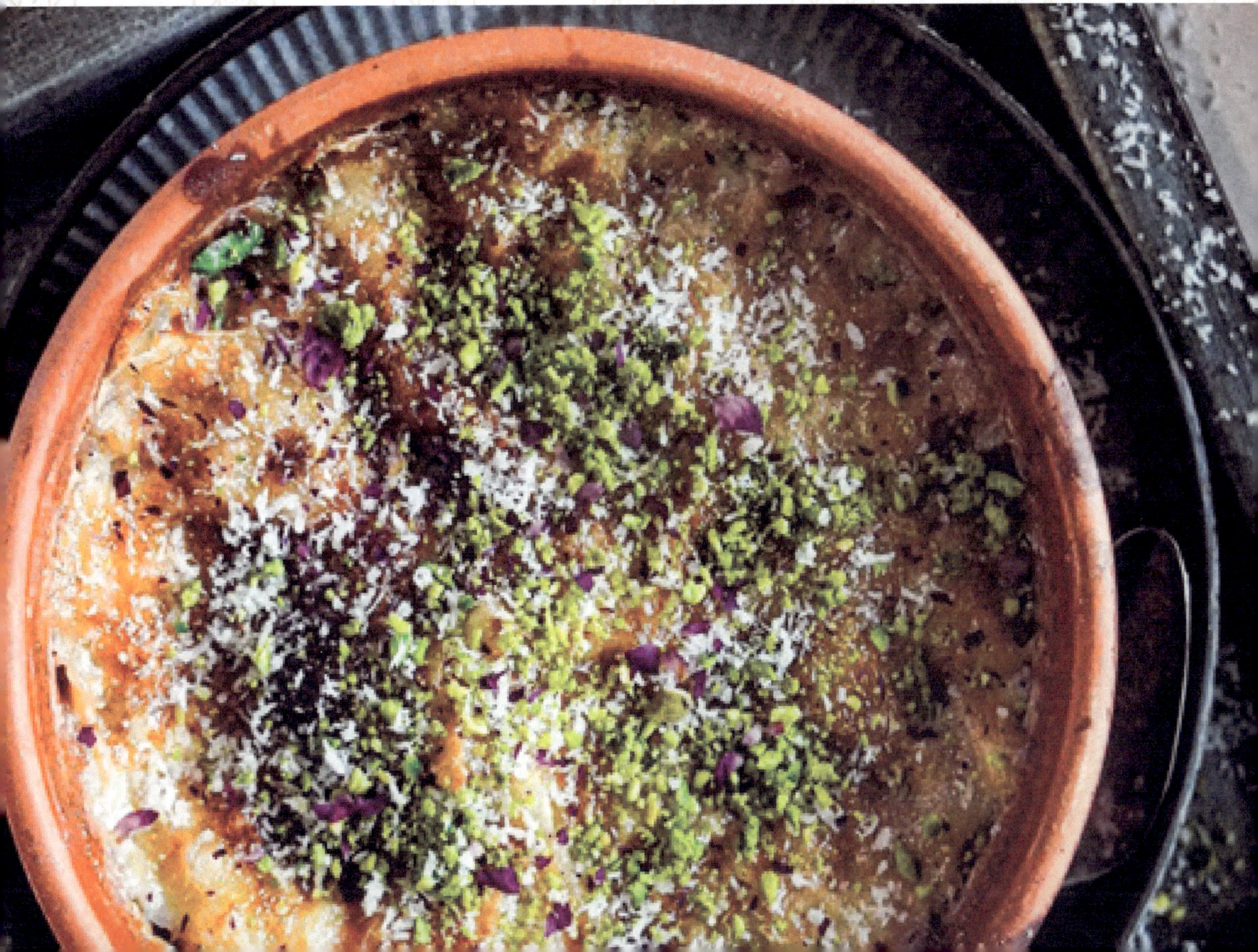

Warbat Bil Qishta وربات بالقشطة

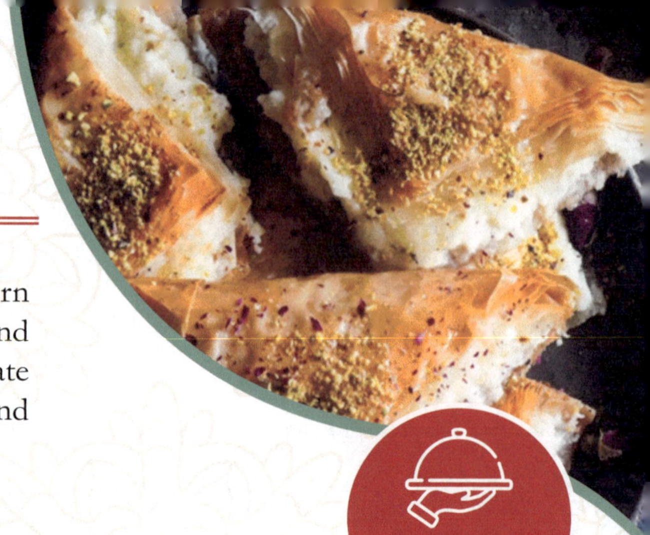

Warbat, also known as Shaabiya, is a delectable Middle Eastern pastry that's enjoyed particularly during special occasions and plenty during Ramadan. This sweet treat is known for its delicate layers of thin phyllo pastry dough that's stuffed with a creamy and cheesy qishta filling.

SERVES

INGREDIENTS:

Warbat:

- 1lb phyllo dough (454g)
- 5 tbsp unsalted butter
- 3 tbsp ghee

Filling:

- Qishta Arabiya

Qater (simple syrup):

- 3 cups granulated sugar
- 2 cups water
- 1 tbsp lemon juice
- 1 tsp orange blossom water

DIRECTIONS:

1. Prepare the simple syrup. Start by combining the granulated sugar and water in a pot, and place them on high heat. Let the mixture come to a boil.
2. Once boiled for 10 minutes, add in the lemon juice and the orange blossom water.
3. Stir, and set aside to cool completely at room temperature.
4. Preheat oven to 350 F.
5. Thaw the phyllo dough according to package instructions.
6. Prepare the Qishta (See Qishta Arabiya recipe).
7. Melt the butter.
8. Begin by rolling out the phyllo dough. Count the sheets, and divide them in half. (My package had 30 sheets, so I divided them into two sets of 15).
9. Lay your first half set of sheets into a flat rectangle. Cut each rectangle into 9 or 12 equal sized squares.

10. Add about 2 tablespoons of qishta in the center of each square, then fold over 1 sheet of dough from the opposite corner of the square to form a triangle shape.
11. Now, fold over two sheets from the top corner of the square to make a triangle shape that holds the qishta in the middle.
12. Brush the top with melted butter, and repeat every two sheets until the triangle shape is fully complete. Repeat until all the phyllo is filled and buttered.
13. Prep a cookie sheet and brush it with the ghee.
14. Add the filled warbat triangles to the tray and let them air dry for an hour. This helps them retain their crunch.
15. Bake at 350 F for about 25-35 minutes, or until the bottom and the top are golden brown. Do not over bake.
16. Once out of the oven, immediately pour the simple syrup on top. Each piece needs about 2-4 tablespoons, depending on desired sweetness.
17. Garnish with finely chopped pistachios and let it cool before serving.

Pro Tip: Do not overfill the warbat. The filling will leak out and you'll have an empty phyllo triangle at the end.

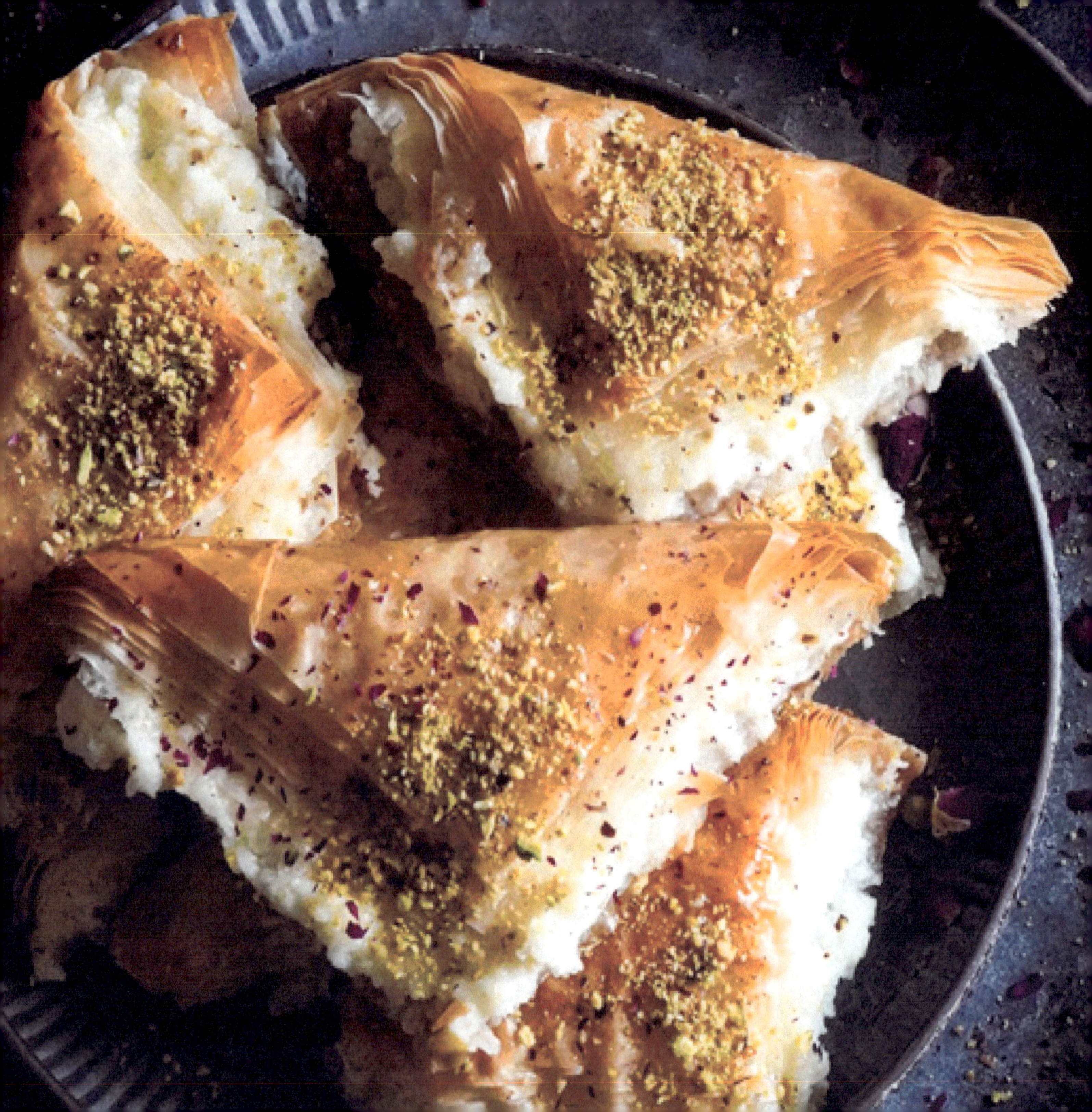

Znoud El Sit زنود الست

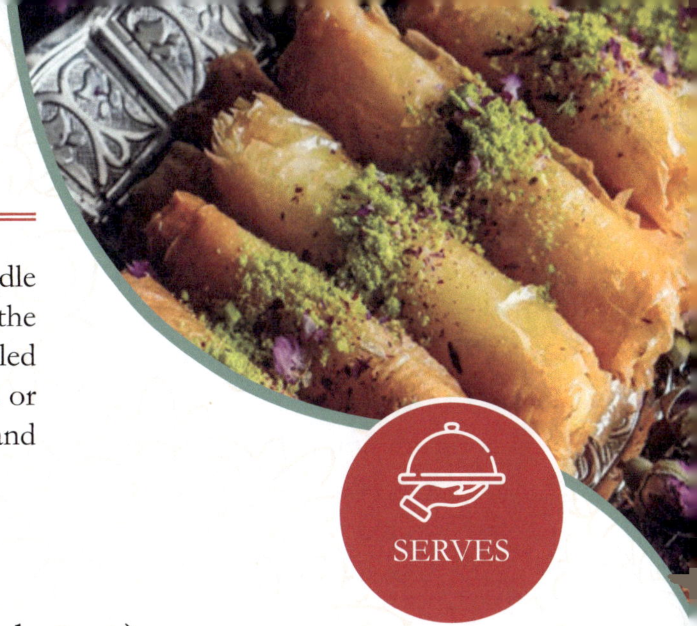

Znoud El Sit, translated as "Lady Arms," is a delectable Middle Eastern dessert that hails from Lebanon and is popular across the region. This sweet treat is characterized by its thin, rolled pastry filled with a creamy mixture, often containing ingredients like custard or clotted cream. Znoud El Sit is then deep-fried until golden and crispy before being generously coated in sugar syrup.

INGREDIENTS:

Creamy Custard Filling:

- 3 cups heavy whipping cream
- 4 tbsp cornstarch
- 1 tsp orange blossom water
- ½ cup granulated sugar
- Phyllo dough sheets
- Neutral oil, for frying

Qater (simple syrup):

- 3 cups granulated sugar
- 2 cups water
- 1 tbsp lemon juice
- 1 tsp orange blossom water

DIRECTIONS:

Make sure to thaw the phyllo dough according to package instructions.

1. Prepare the simple syrup. Start by combining the granulated sugar and water in a pot, and place them on high heat. Let the mixture come to a boil.
2. Once boiled for 10 minutes, add in the lemon juice and the orange blossom water.
3. Stir, and set aside to cool completely at room temperature.
4. To prepare the filling, combine the heavy whipping cream and cornstarch in a saucepan, without turning on the heat. Whisk well until the cornstarch is dissolved and no longer visible.
5. Add the granulated sugar, and place on medium heat. Whisk well.
6. Continuously whisk for 6-12 minutes, or until the cream has thickened.
7. Add the orange blossom water and give it a quick stir before removing from heat.

8. Transfer the cream to a plate and cover with plastic wrap. Refrigerate until completely cooled.
9. Cut the phyllo dough into 4-inch by 2-inch pieces to make rectangles.
10. Using two sheets at a time, make an upside down T shape.
11. Add cooled cream onto the edge of the T-shaped phyllo sheets.
12. Fold the edges over to cover the cream, then roll up like a cigar.
13. Place a small amount of cream on the edges to help it seal.
14. Let them sit on a plate while heating up the oil on medium-high heat. These need to be deep fried, so use a good amount of oil and a deep pot.
15. Drop the rolled phyllo cigars in and fry until golden brown.
16. Use a slotted spoon to remove the fried cigars, and immediately dip into the simple syrup.
17. Let it sit in the simple syrup for 20-30 seconds before removing. Garnish with ground pistachios.

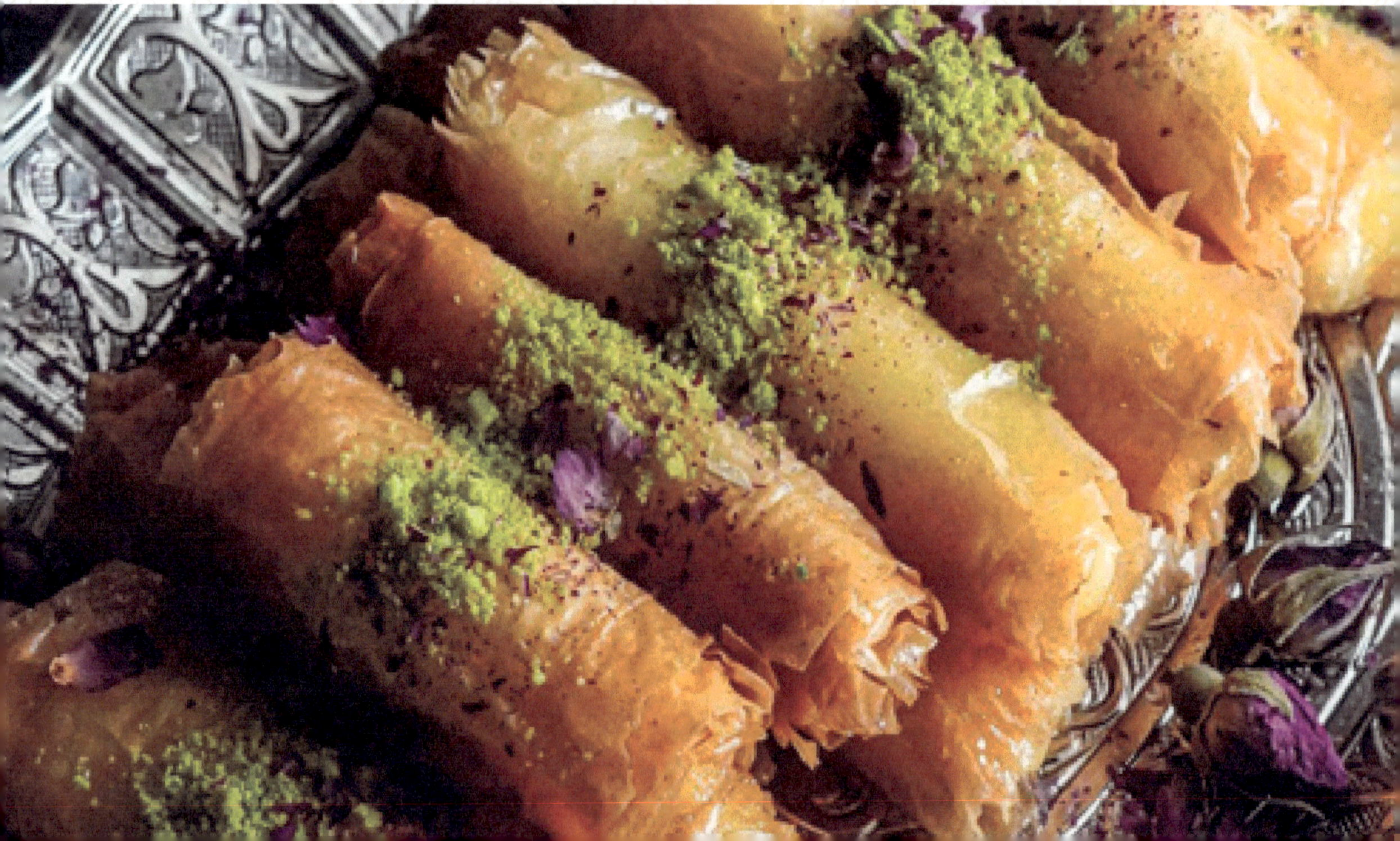

Pistachio Baklawa بقلاوة بالفستق

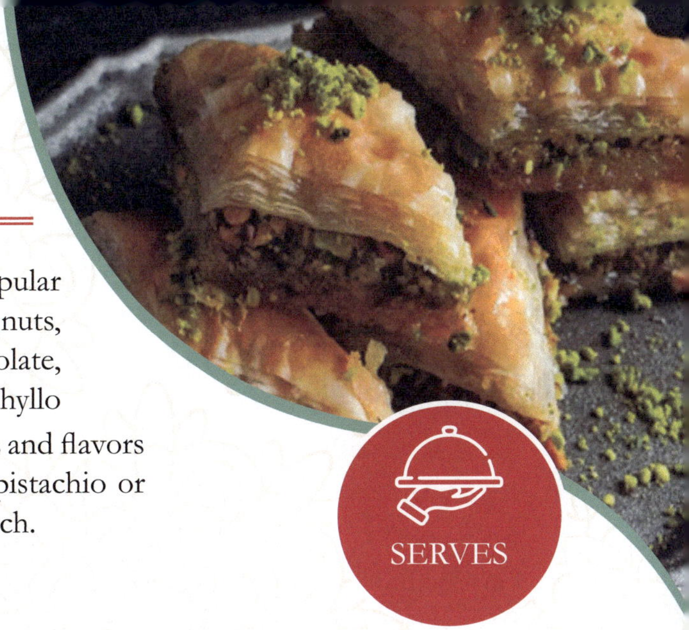

Baklawa, or as some know it, baklava, is one of the most popular desserts across the Middle East. It's filled with different types of nuts, and nowadays, people alter the traditional ingredients to add chocolate, or cookie butter. Multiple layers of crispy, flakey, and buttery phyllo dough with a fragrant pistachio filling form a marriage of textures and flavors that is unforgettable. The most traditional type of baklawa is pistachio or walnut, and in Palestine, usually both are not mixed into one batch.

SERVES

INGREDIENTS:

- 2 ½ cups coarsely chopped unsalted & raw pistachios
- ½ tbsp orange blossom water
- ½ tsp cardamom, ground
- ½ cup granulated sugar
- ½ cup ghee
- ½ cup unsalted butter
- 30-34 sheets of phyllo dough, thawed according to package instructions

Qater (simple syrup):

- 3½ cups sugar
- 2 cups water
- 1½ tsp lemon juice
- 1 tbsp orange blossom water

DIRECTIONS:

*Make the simple syrup ahead of time by combining the water, sugar, and lemon juice on medium high heat. Let it boil for 5 minutes before simmering on medium-low heat for another 10 minutes. Add the orange blossom water now, and let the syrup cool completely before making the baklawa.

1. Preheat the oven to 350 degrees.
2. Thaw the phyllo dough according to package instructions, and prepare the simple syrup ahead of time so it's at room temperature.
3. Coarsely chop the pistachios in the food processor and transfer them to a bowl.
4. Add the sugar, and orange blossom water. Mix well and set aside.

5. Melt the ghee and butter in a bowl and set aside.
6. Count the phyllo dough sheets in the package. We are looking for 30-34 sheets. The Athens brand has two divided wrapped phyllo dough sheets per 1 pound package, which makes it easy to use.
7. Brush 1 tablespoon of the butter and ghee mixture onto your 9*13 pan. Trim about ½ inch to ¾ inch of the phyllo dough from the short side to make it fit the pan. You can also use a slightly bigger pan without trimming. Place 3 sheets of phyllo at a time, flat, then lightly brush with the ghee and butter mixture. Repeat until half the amount of sheets are finished. Place the pistachio mixture on top evenly.
8. Now, lay another 2 phyllo sheets on top and lightly brush with butter/ ghee mixture. Place another 3 sheets and repeat. For the last sheet, lightly brush.You should have some ghee/ butter leftover, about □ to ½ cup.
9. Cut the baklawa into your desired shape, making sure to cut all the way to the bottom.
10. Pour the remaining amount of butter and ghee all over, so it gets through the cuts.
11. Place in the oven at 350 F for about 50-55 minutes, until it gets golden. You can rotate the pan halfway to make sure it browns evenly. Once out of the oven, immediately pour the room temperature syrup on top.
12. Garnish with finely chopped pistachios (if desired) and place into the fridge to cool for 2-3 hours.Once cooled, reinforce the cuts again. Let it come to room temperature before removing and serving. Do not cover.

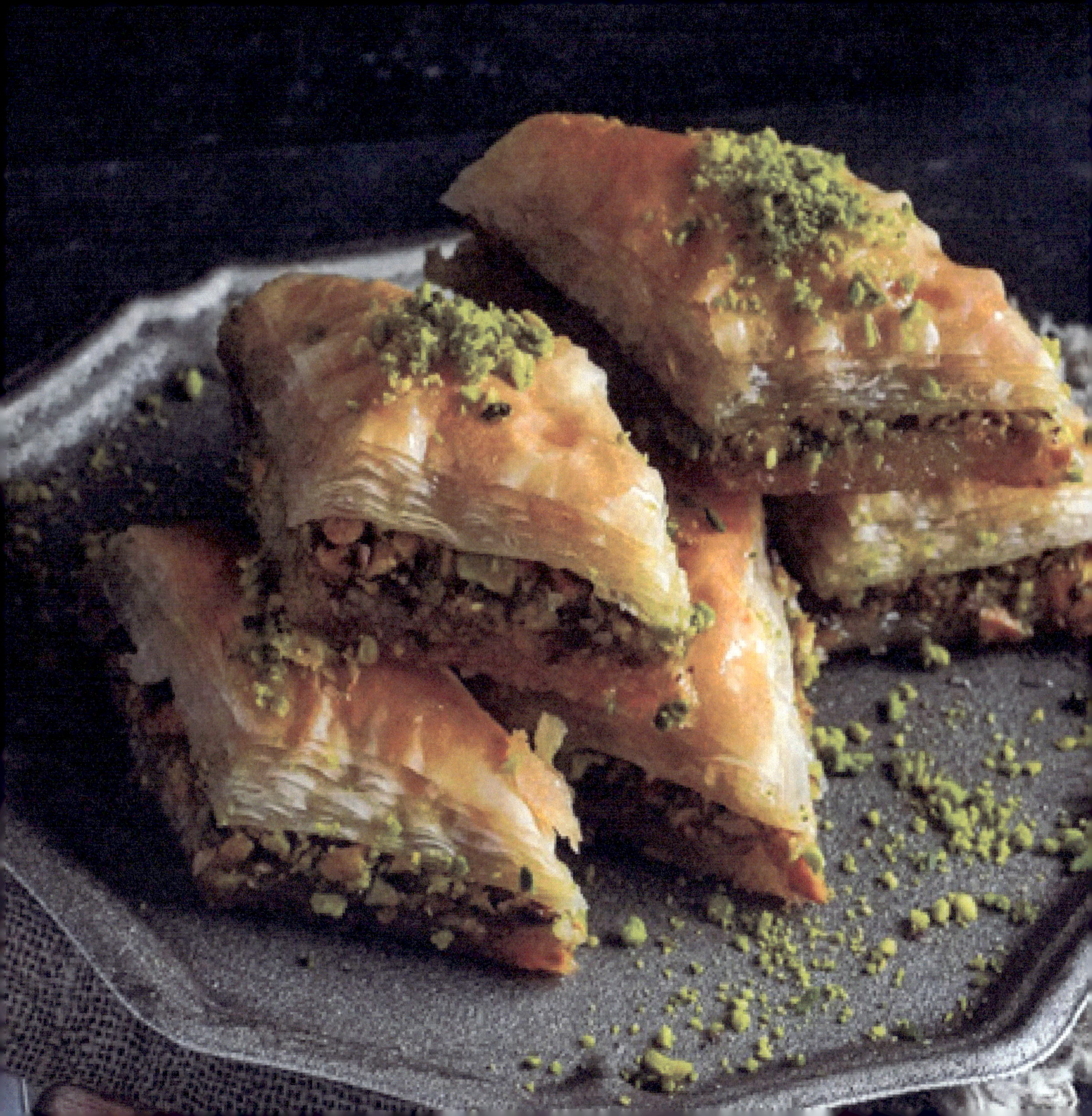

Booza Arabiya بوظة عربية

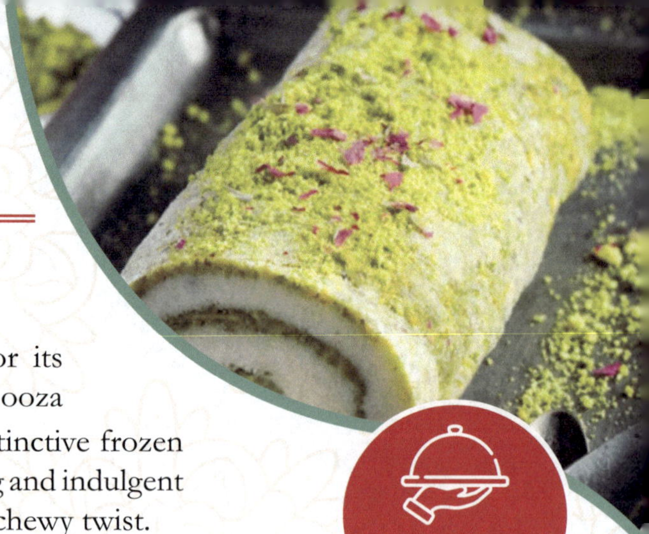

(Middle Eastern Ice cream)

Booza, a traditional Middle Eastern ice cream, stands out for its unique texture and rich, dense flavor. Unlike regular ice cream, Booza is known for its chewy and stretchy consistency, making it a distinctive frozen treat. Whether served in a cone or a bowl, Booza offers a satisfying and indulgent experience, combining the creamy richness of ice cream with a chewy twist.

MAKES
1 large bowl

INGREDIENTS:

- 3 cups whole milk
- 3 ⅓ cups heavy whipping cream
- 2 tbsp + ⅛ tsp pure salep powder
- ¾ tsp crushed mastic rocks
- 1 cup + 2 tbsp granulated sugar
- ½ tsp orange blossom water
- 2 cups finely chopped pistachios

DIRECTIONS:

1. Put the mastic with a small pinch of sugar and crush using a mortar and pestle. Make sure no large chunks remain and it's completely ground.
2. Add the milk, heavy whipping cream, salep powder, and sugar to a sauce pan on medium heat. Add the crushed mastic.
3. Mix everything well, and whisk often on medium heat until ribbons begin falling from the spoon, about 20 minutes.
4. Once ribbons begin forming, add in the orange blossom water.
5. Remove and set aside to cool for 20 minutes at room temperature.
6. Once cooled, pour the mixture into a bowl of a stand mixer. Using the whisk attachment, whisk everything for about 5 minutes.
7. Cover the bowl with plastic wrap and freeze for 2 hours.
8. Now, return to the stand mixer and whisk again for another 5 minutes.
9. Cover with plastic wrap and freeze for another 2 hours, once again.

10. Now, transfer to the standmixer once again, and blend with the whisk attachment for another 5 minutes.
11. In the meantime, line a cookie sheet with plastic wrap. Add the crushed pistachios over it. Pour the blended cream mix on top, and cover with more plastic wrap. Freeze for another 1-2 hours. You want this to be thick, but not brick solid. If it's too soft, it won't roll properly. If it's too thick, it'll break as you roll it. It needs to be semi-frozen.
12. Once semi-frozen, remove the top plastic wrap layer. Take the bottom plastic wrap (the one you lined the cookie sheet with) and begin slowly wrapping it like you would a swiss roll. Careful to only use the plastic as guidance, and to not roll it into the actual ice cream.
13. Once completely rolled, cover with plastic and freeze once more for a minimum of 4 hours. Once completely frozen, wrap with aluminum foil to preserve freshness.

Pro Tips:

» If you messed up on the rolling, don't fret. Just add it to a container and scoop it using an ice cream scoop.

» It's important to use pure salep powder to give it that authentic stretch.

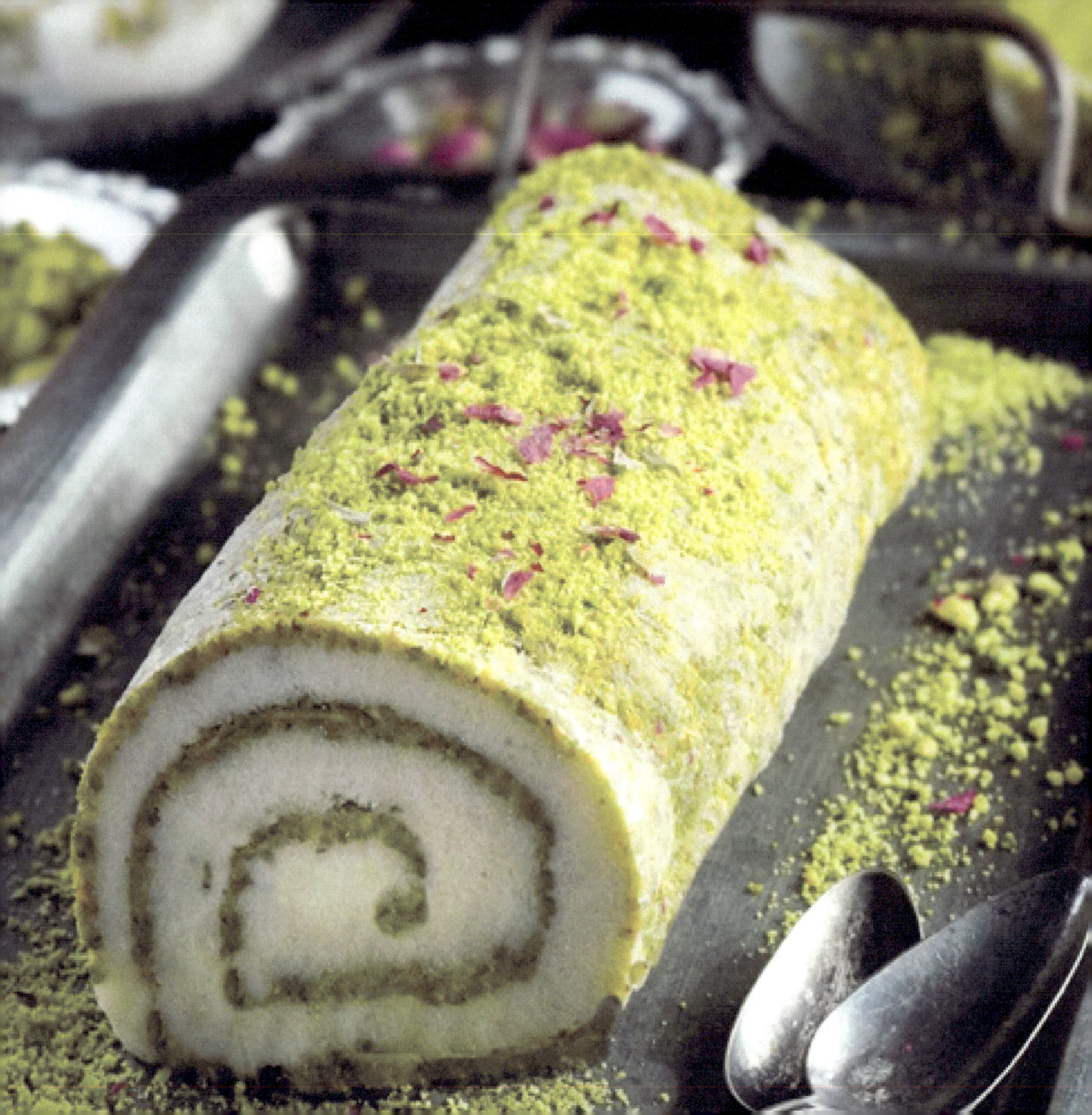

Yemeni Adeni Shai شاي عدني

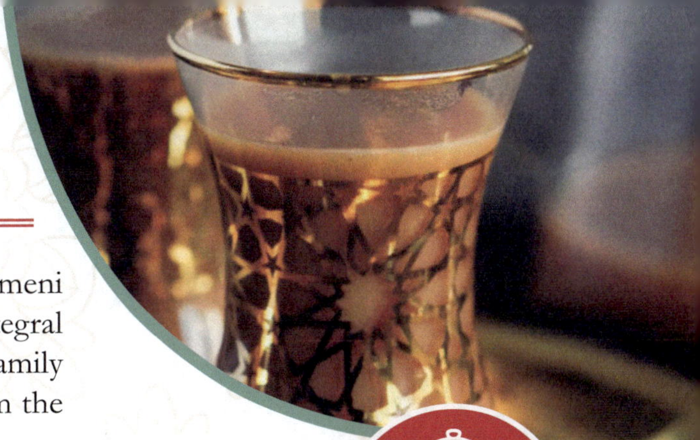

Adeni tea, also known as Adeni chai, is a popular and aromatic Yemeni tea with a distinctive flavor profile. This traditional tea is an integral part of Yemeni culture and is often enjoyed in social gatherings, family settings, and during various occasions. The tea could differ from the spices used to the amounts according to each person's liking.

SERVES 4

INGREDIENTS:

- 4½ cups water
- 2 tbsp granulated sugar, or to taste
- 1 tsp ground cardamom
- Pinch of nutmeg
- 2 whole cloves
- 4 black tea bags or 2 tablespoons loose black tea
- ½ cup evaporated milk

DIRECTIONS:

1. Mix the water and sugar into a teapot.
2. Add the tea bags or loose tea and the spices, and let it boil for 5 minutes on high heat.
3. Turn off the heat and let it steep another 5-8 minutes.
4. Remove the tea bags or loose tea and the whole spices.
5. Add in the evaporated milk and mix.
6. Return to the stove for another 3-5 minutes on medium low until fully heated and bubbly.
7. Remove and serve with some more sugar to taste.

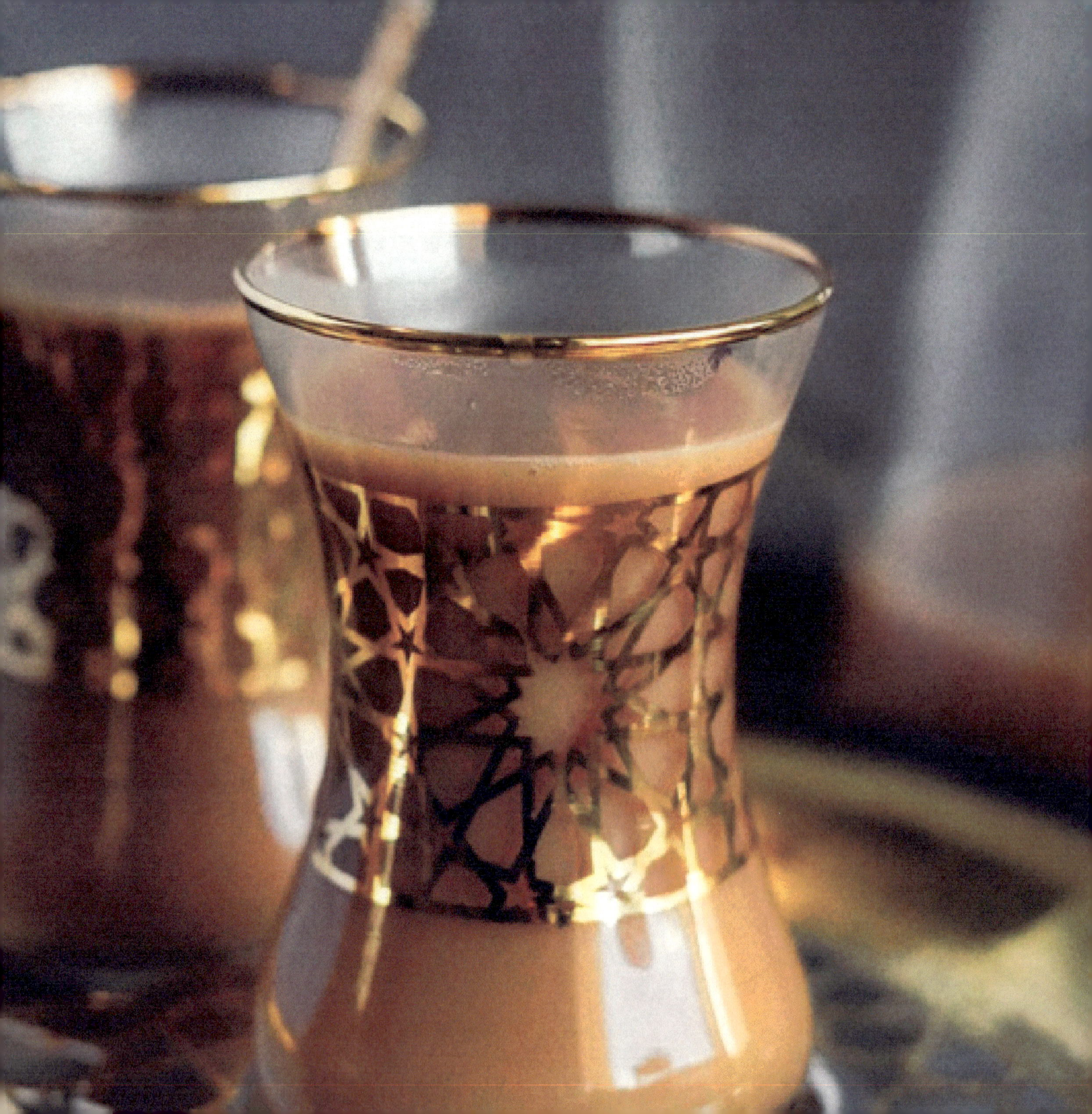

Pomegranate Spritzer

مشروب الرمان

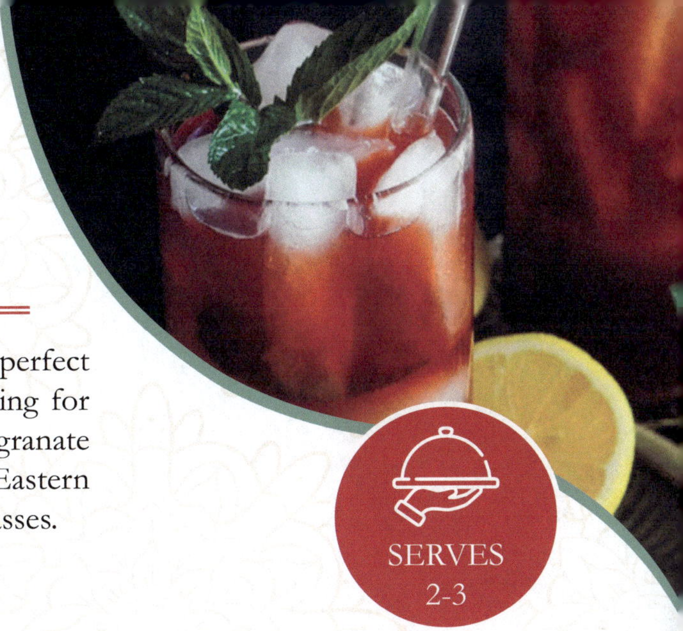

This spritzer is a refreshing and easy-to-make drink that strikes the perfect balance between sweet and tangy flavors. Whether you're looking for a quick pick-me-up or a delightful hosting beverage, this Pomegranate Spritzer is a great go-to choice. It utilizes commonly used Middle Eastern ingredients like mint, lemon-lime flavors, and pomegranate molasses.

SERVES 2-3

INGREDIENTS:

- 3 cups lemon-lime flavored soda
- ½ cup pomegranate juice
- ½ cup mint leaves
- ½ cup cold water
- 3 tbsp pomegranate molasses
- Ice

DIRECTIONS:

1. Start by tearing the mint leaves by hand, avoiding chopping them. This ensures they release the oils without losing the flavor on a cutting board or knife. Add them to a large pitcher.
2. Drizzle in the 3 tablespoons of pomegranate molasses. Use a pestle to lightly muddle them together.
3. Add the ½ cup cold water, the ½ cup pomegranate juice, and the 3 cups soda. Stir well with a large spoon or ladle.
4. Add enough ice to keep everything cool and refreshing, about 2-3 cups. Stir, and serve with more mint leaves and lemon wedges.

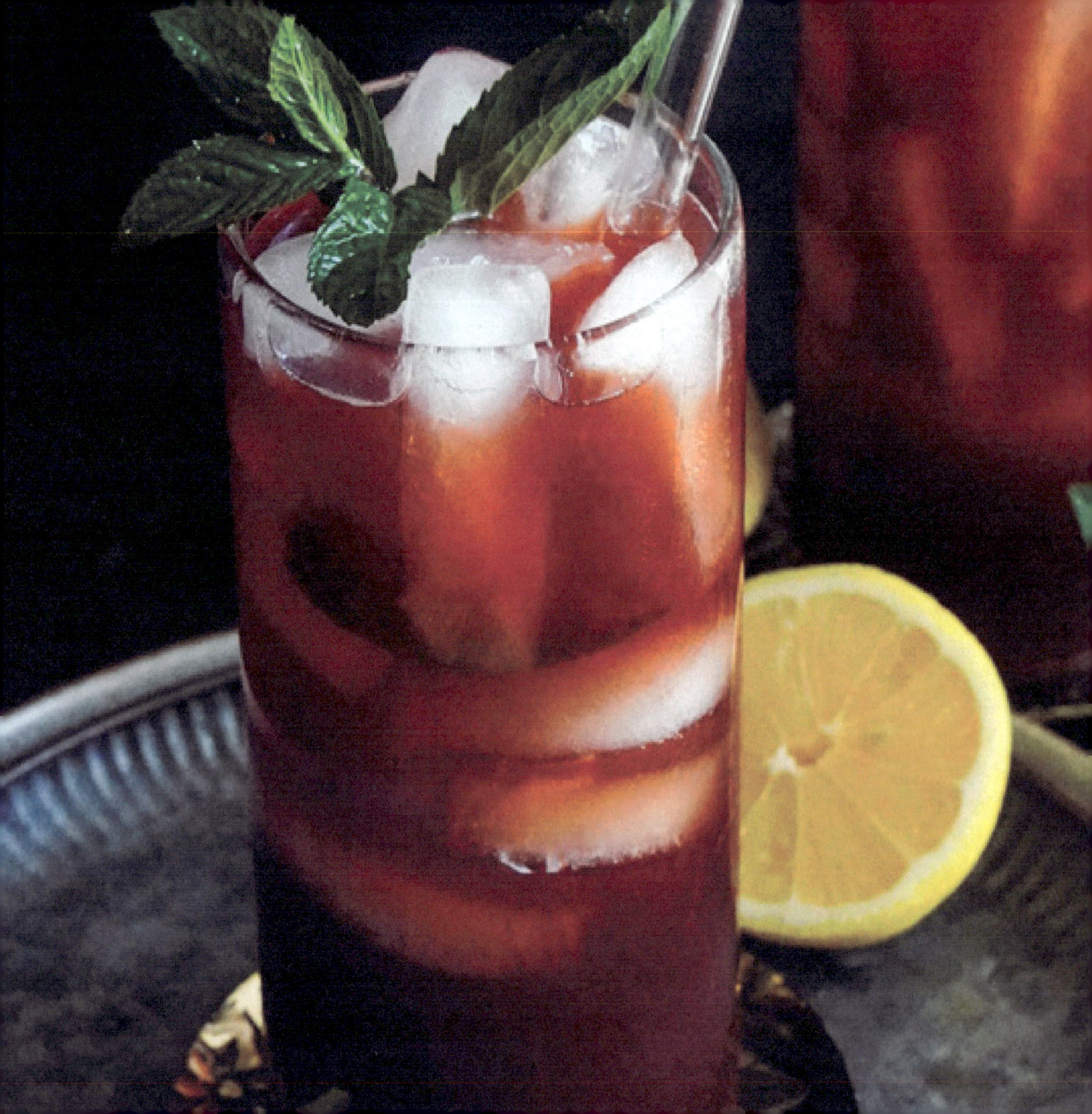

Sahlab سحلب

Sahlab, also spelled Salep, is a customary Middle Eastern and Mediterranean hot beverage known for its comforting and creamy texture. It is particularly popular during the winter months and is enjoyed as a warm and soothing drink. Muslims also often enjoy it during Ramadan after iftar or for suhoor.

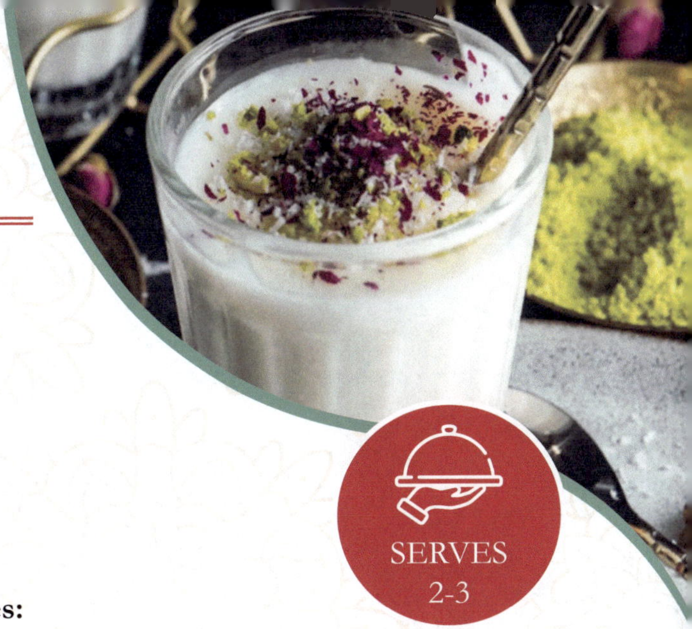

SERVES 2-3

INGREDIENTS:

Sahlab:

- 3 cups whole milk
- 1 tsp orange blossom or rose water
- 1/4 cup granulated sugar (or to taste)
- 2 tbsp cornstarch
- 2 mastic rocks, finely crushed (if available)

Garnishes:

- Pistachio
- Almonds
- Coconut
- Cinnamon
- Edible rose petals

DIRECTIONS:

1. Add all the ingredients to a saucepan, without turning on the stove. Mix to make sure the cornstarch is fully dissolved and not chunky.
2. Add the saucepan to the stove on medium heat, stirring constantly.
3. Stir until thickened, about 5-10 minutes.
4. Transfer to cups or bowls and garnish.

Pro Tip: Sahlab is a drink, but it could also be made thicker to be eaten with a spoon. If you prefer that consistency, add more cornstarch.

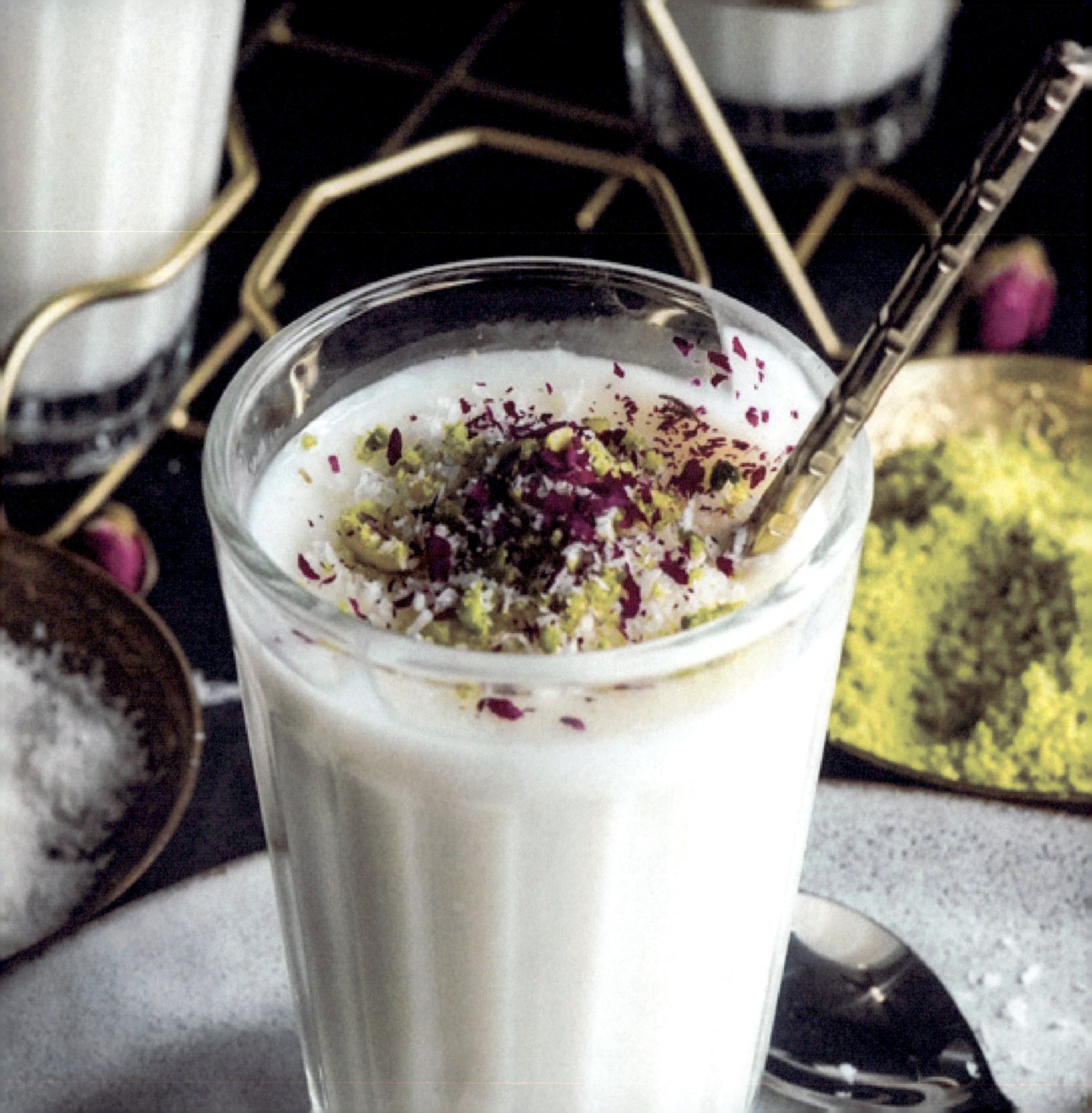

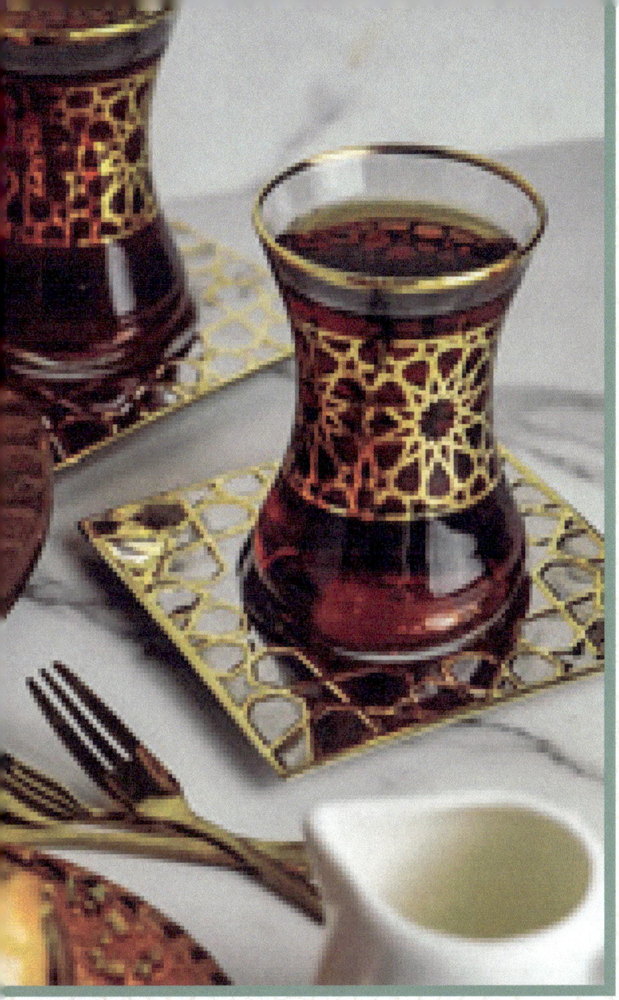
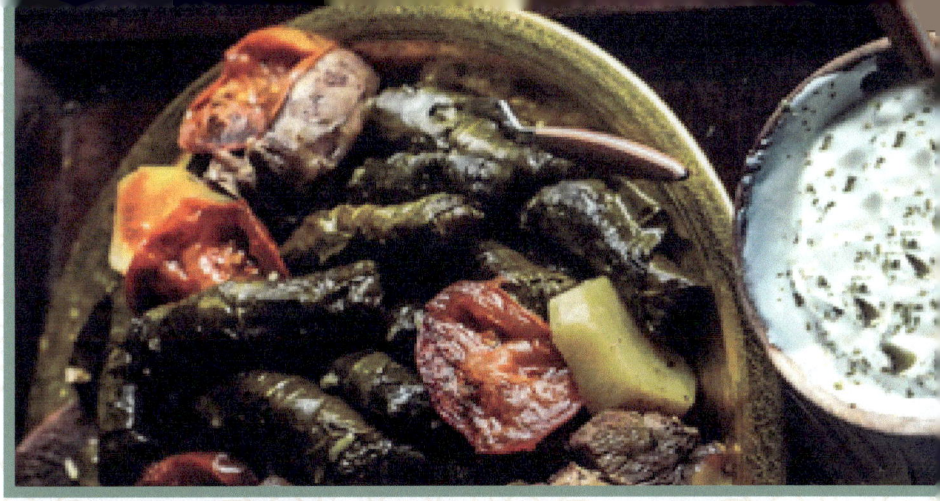
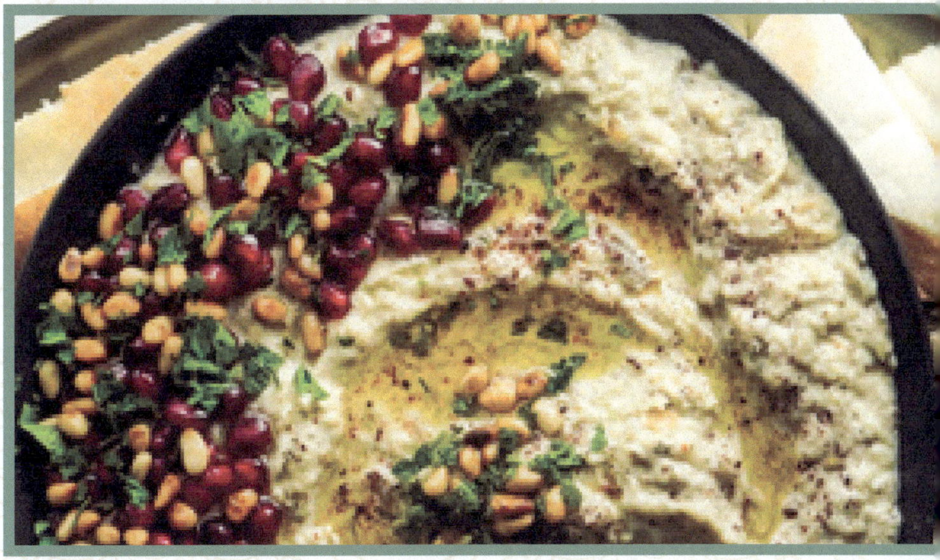
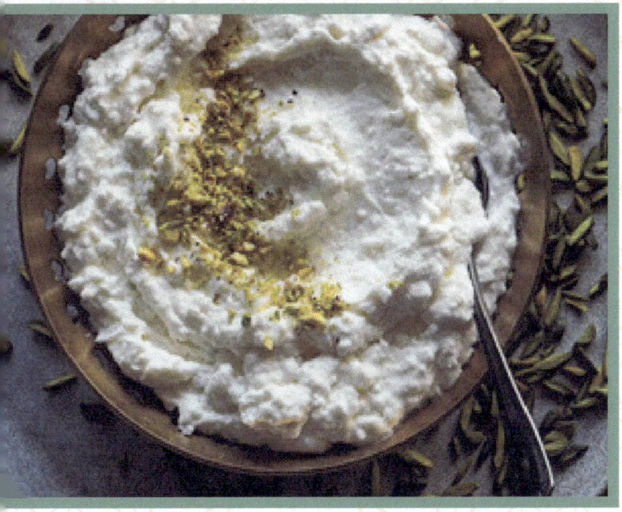
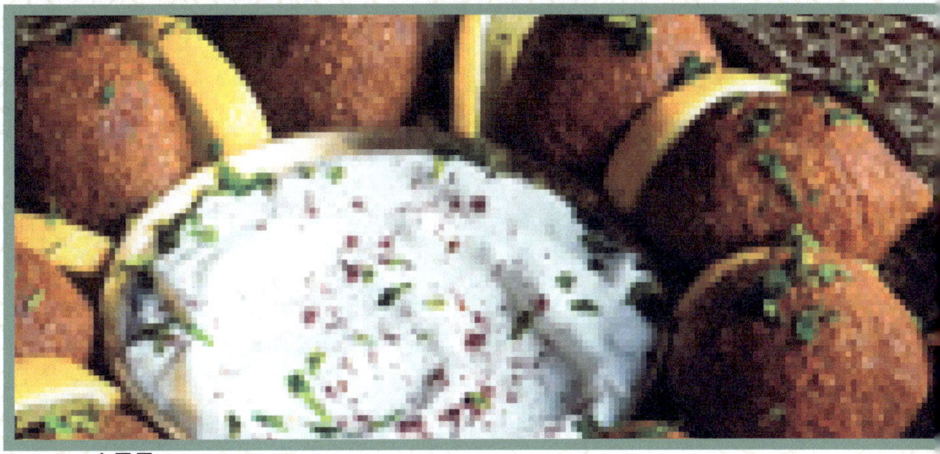

Acknowledgements

All Praise is due to The Most High, the Most Merciful. “This is by the Grace of My Lord” (27:40).

To my husband: Thank you for always supporting me in all my cooking adventures and endeavors. This book would have never been possible without all of your encouragement and your constant push to make me reach my full potential.

To my mom: Thank you for always supporting my content creation even though you don’t believe in the use of measuring spoons or cups. Thank you for making such great food that it inspired me to share your recipes with everyone on the internet (everyone LOVES them!)

To my soul-sister Leen: Thank you for always listening to me when I needed to vent about my work. Thank you for being there despite the distance.

To the instagram friends that became family: Thank you for your constant duas, and for your endless support. You all had a lot on your own plates but still gave me immense support and advice. I ask God to bless you in all your endeavors and to grant you immense happiness.

To my two little boys: I love you, and ask God to keep you safe and happy.

To my Falasteenifoodie instagram family: Thank you for all the countless support on this four year journey. It’s been tough, and I wouldn’t have been able to do this without you and your constant support.

To you, the reader: Thank you for giving me a chance, and thank you for supporting me. I hope you benefit from it and enjoy it fully.

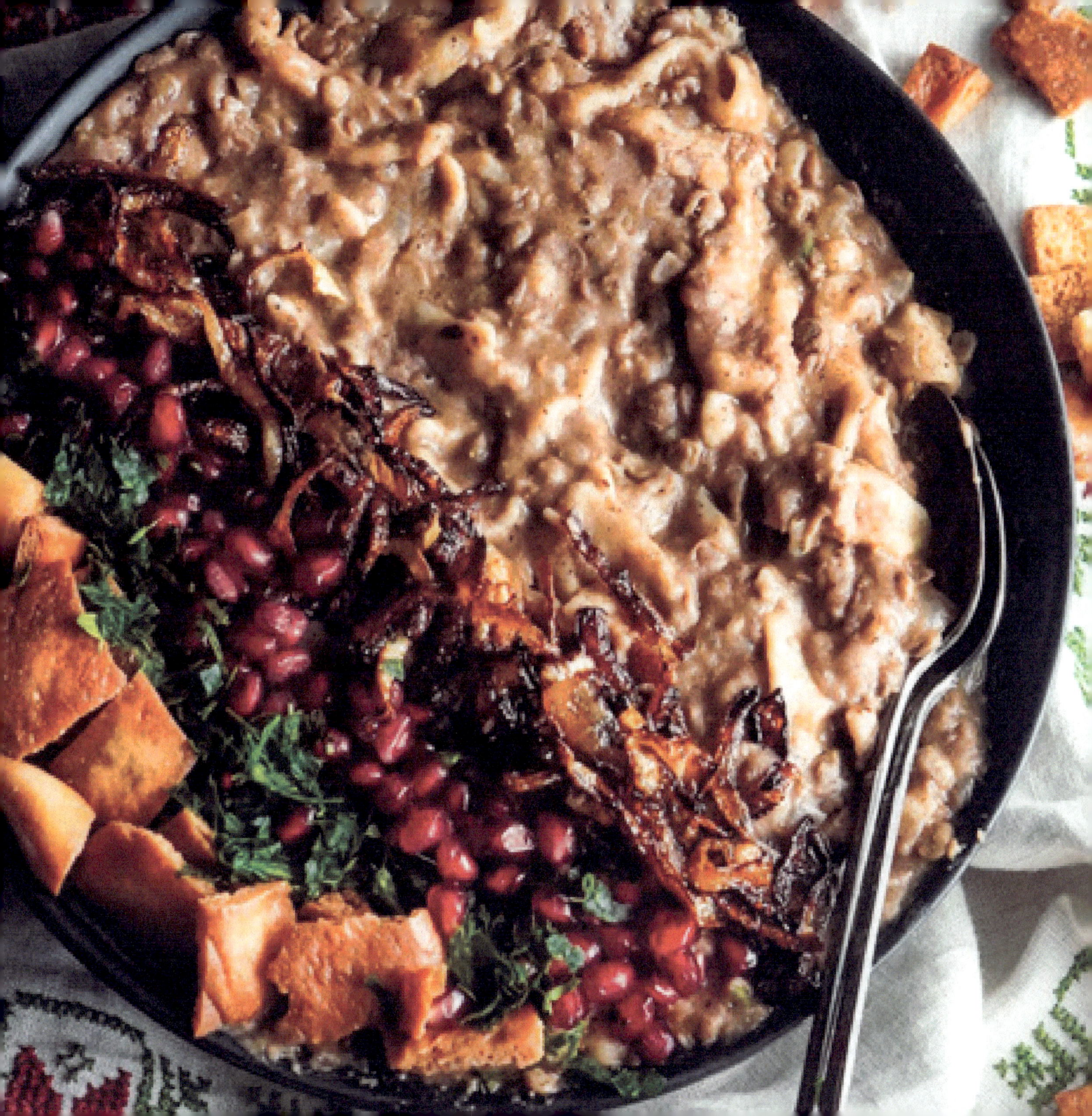

About the Author

Fatimah M.A. is a first generation Palestinian-American. A food blogger, food enthusiast, wife and a mother of two, her journey began with documenting her recipes and cooking in order to feel a connection to Palestine and Arabs across all diasporas. She's adamant about trying new cultural dishes and traditions from across the globe, and hopes to spread her love for them to every corner of the globe. She hopes that by sharing delicious recipes from Arab countries that it'll help reshape the narrative about Arabs and their cultures, one bite at a time.

You can follow Fatimah's food and recipe journeys on her blog at

falasteenifoodie.com

or watch her recipe videos on Instagram and TikTok

@falasteenifoodie.

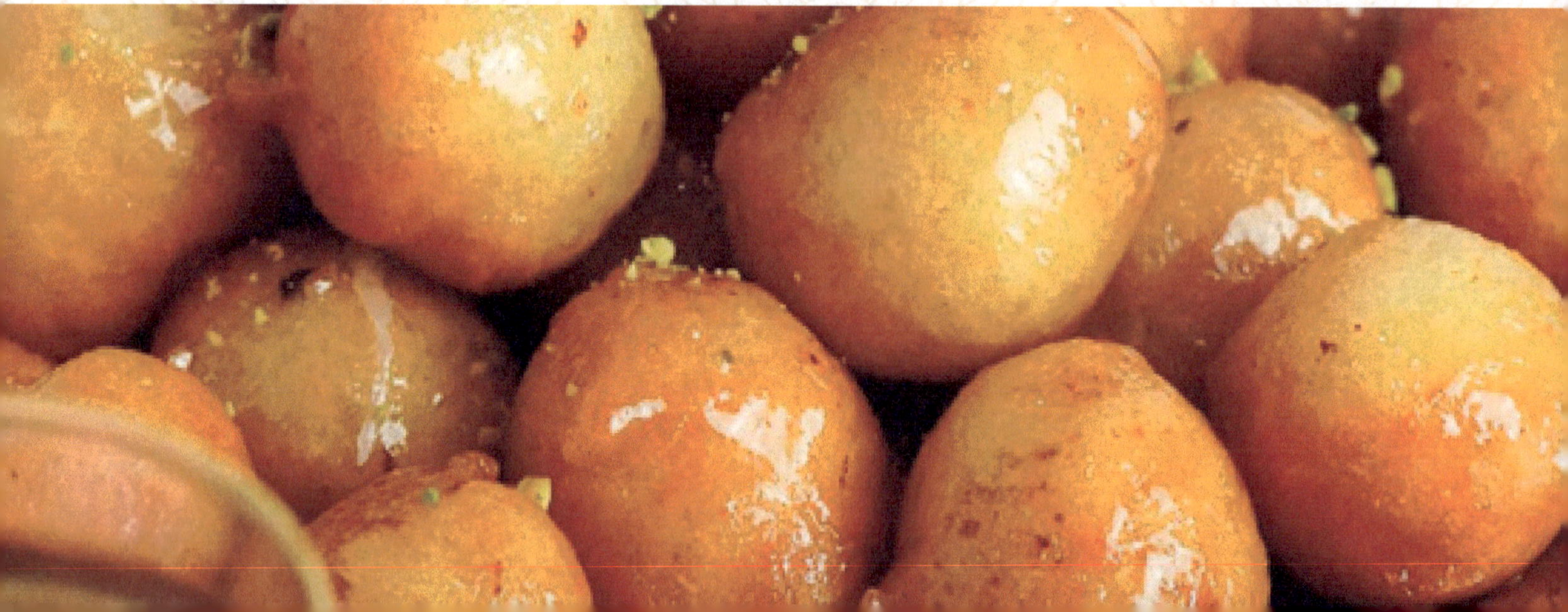

Printed in France by Amazon
Brétigny-sur-Orge, FR

18714184R00089